OSTEOPATHY

A MEDICAL DICTIONARY, BIBLIOGRAPHY,
AND ANNOTATED RESEARCH GUIDE TO
INTERNET REFERENCES

JAMES N. PARKER, M.D.
AND PHILIP M. PARKER, PH.D., EDITORS

ii

ICON Health Publications
ICON Group International, Inc.
4370 La Jolla Village Drive, 4th Floor
San Diego, CA 92122 USA

Printed in the United States of America.

Last digit indicates print number: 10 9 8 7 6 4 5 3 2 1

Publisher, Health Care: Philip Parker, Ph.D.
Editor(s): James Parker, M.D., Philip Parker, Ph.D.

Publisher's note: The ideas, procedures, and suggestions contained in this book are not intended for the diagnosis or treatment of a health problem. As new medical or scientific information becomes available from academic and clinical research, recommended treatments and drug therapies may undergo changes. The authors, editors, and publisher have attempted to make the information in this book up to date and accurate in accord with accepted standards at the time of publication. The authors, editors, and publisher are not responsible for errors or omissions or for consequences from application of the book, and make no warranty, expressed or implied, in regard to the contents of this book. Any practice described in this book should be applied by the reader in accordance with professional standards of care used in regard to the unique circumstances that may apply in each situation. The reader is advised to always check product information (package inserts) for changes and new information regarding dosage and contraindications before prescribing any drug or pharmacological product. Caution is especially urged when using new or infrequently ordered drugs, herbal remedies, vitamins and supplements, alternative therapies, complementary therapies and medicines, and integrative medical treatments.

Cataloging-in-Publication Data

Parker, James N., 1961-
Parker, Philip M., 1960-

    Osteopathy: A Medical Dictionary, Bibliography, and Annotated Research Guide to Internet References / James N. Parker and Philip M. Parker, editors
             p.   cm.
    Includes bibliographical references, glossary, and index.
    ISBN: 0-497-00811-4
    1. Osteopathy-Popular works.   I. Title.

Disclaimer

This publication is not intended to be used for the diagnosis or treatment of a health problem. It is sold with the understanding that the publisher, editors, and authors are not engaging in the rendering of medical, psychological, financial, legal, or other professional services.

References to any entity, product, service, or source of information that may be contained in this publication should not be considered an endorsement, either direct or implied, by the publisher, editors, or authors. ICON Group International, Inc., the editors, and the authors are not responsible for the content of any Web pages or publications referenced in this publication.

Copyright Notice

Acknowledgements

The collective knowledge generated from academic and applied research summarized in various references has been critical in the creation of this book which is best viewed as a comprehensive compilation and collection of information prepared by various official agencies which produce publications on osteopathy. Books in this series draw from various agencies and institutions associated with the United States Department of Health and Human Services, and in particular, the Office of the Secretary of Health and Human Services (OS), the Administration for Children and Families (ACF), the Administration on Aging (AOA), the Agency for Healthcare Research and Quality (AHRQ), the Agency for Toxic Substances and Disease Registry (ATSDR), the Centers for Disease Control and Prevention (CDC), the Food and Drug Administration (FDA), the Healthcare Financing Administration (HCFA), the Health Resources and Services Administration (HRSA), the Indian Health Service (IHS), the institutions of the National Institutes of Health (NIH), the Program Support Center (PSC), and the Substance Abuse and Mental Health Services Administration (SAMHSA). In addition to these sources, information gathered from the National Library of Medicine, the United States Patent Office, the European Union, and their related organizations has been invaluable in the creation of this book. Some of the work represented was financially supported by the Research and Development Committee at INSEAD. This support is gratefully acknowledged. Finally, special thanks are owed to Tiffany Freeman for her excellent editorial support.

About the Editors

James N. Parker, M.D.

Dr. James N. Parker received his Bachelor of Science degree in Psychobiology from the University of California, Riverside and his M.D. from the University of California, San Diego. In addition to authoring numerous research publications, he has lectured at various academic institutions. Dr. Parker is the medical editor for health books by ICON Health Publications.

Philip M. Parker, Ph.D.

Philip M. Parker is the Eli Lilly Chair Professor of Innovation, Business and Society at INSEAD (Fontainebleau, France and Singapore). Dr. Parker has also been Professor at the University of California, San Diego and has taught courses at Harvard University, the Hong Kong University of Science and Technology, the Massachusetts Institute of Technology, Stanford University, and UCLA. Dr. Parker is the associate editor for ICON Health Publications.

About ICON Health Publications

To discover more about ICON Health Publications, simply check with your preferred online booksellers, including Barnes&Noble.com and Amazon.com which currently carry all of our titles. Or, feel free to contact us directly for bulk purchases or institutional discounts:

ICON Group International, Inc.
4370 La Jolla Village Drive, Fourth Floor
San Diego, CA 92122 USA
Fax: 858-546-4341
Web site: **www.icongrouponline.com/health**

Table of Contents

FORWARD 1
CHAPTER 1. STUDIES ON OSTEOPATHY 3
    Overview 3
    The Combined Health Information Database 3
    Federally Funded Research on Osteopathy 4
    E-Journals: PubMed Central 6
    The National Library of Medicine: PubMed 6
CHAPTER 2. NUTRITION AND OSTEOPATHY 23
    Overview 23
    Finding Nutrition Studies on Osteopathy 23
    Federal Resources on Nutrition 24
    Additional Web Resources 24
CHAPTER 3. ALTERNATIVE MEDICINE AND OSTEOPATHY 27
    Overview 27
    The Combined Health Information Database 27
    National Center for Complementary and Alternative Medicine 28
    Additional Web Resources 29
    General References 31
CHAPTER 4. PATENTS ON OSTEOPATHY 33
    Overview 33
    Patents on Osteopathy 33
    Patent Applications on Osteopathy 34
    Keeping Current 36
CHAPTER 5. BOOKS ON OSTEOPATHY 39
    Overview 39
    Book Summaries: Federal Agencies 39
    Book Summaries: Online Booksellers 40
APPENDIX A. PHYSICIAN RESOURCES 43
    Overview 43
    NIH Guidelines 43
    NIH Databases 45
    Other Commercial Databases 47
APPENDIX B. PATIENT RESOURCES 49
    Overview 49
    Patient Guideline Sources 49
    Finding Associations 51
APPENDIX C. FINDING MEDICAL LIBRARIES 53
    Overview 53
    Preparation 53
    Finding a Local Medical Library 53
    Medical Libraries in the U.S. and Canada 53

ONLINE GLOSSARIES 59

    Online Dictionary Directories 59

OSTEOPATHY DICTIONARY 61

INDEX 75

FORWARD

In March 2001, the National Institutes of Health issued the following warning: "The number of Web sites offering health-related resources grows every day. Many sites provide valuable information, while others may have information that is unreliable or misleading."[1] Furthermore, because of the rapid increase in Internet-based information, many hours can be wasted searching, selecting, and printing. Since only the smallest fraction of information dealing with osteopathy is indexed in search engines, such as **www.google.com** or others, a non-systematic approach to Internet research can be not only time consuming, but also incomplete. This book was created for medical professionals, students, and members of the general public who want to know as much as possible about osteopathy, using the most advanced research tools available and spending the least amount of time doing so.

In addition to offering a structured and comprehensive bibliography, the pages that follow will tell you where and how to find reliable information covering virtually all topics related to osteopathy, from the essentials to the most advanced areas of research. Public, academic, government, and peer-reviewed research studies are emphasized. Various abstracts are reproduced to give you some of the latest official information available to date on osteopathy. Abundant guidance is given on how to obtain free-of-charge primary research results via the Internet. **While this book focuses on the field of medicine, when some sources provide access to non-medical information relating to osteopathy, these are noted in the text.**

E-book and electronic versions of this book are fully interactive with each of the Internet sites mentioned (clicking on a hyperlink automatically opens your browser to the site indicated). If you are using the hard copy version of this book, you can access a cited Web site by typing the provided Web address directly into your Internet browser. You may find it useful to refer to synonyms or related terms when accessing these Internet databases. **NOTE:** At the time of publication, the Web addresses were functional. However, some links may fail due to URL address changes, which is a common occurrence on the Internet.

For readers unfamiliar with the Internet, detailed instructions are offered on how to access electronic resources. For readers unfamiliar with medical terminology, a comprehensive glossary is provided. For readers without access to Internet resources, a directory of medical libraries, that have or can locate references cited here, is given. We hope these resources will prove useful to the widest possible audience seeking information on osteopathy.

The Editors

---

[1] From the NIH, National Cancer Institute (NCI): **http://www.cancer.gov/cancerinfo/ten-things-to-know**.

Chapter 1. Studies on Osteopathy

Overview

In this chapter, we will show you how to locate peer-reviewed references and studies on osteopathy.

The Combined Health Information Database

The Combined Health Information Database summarizes studies across numerous federal agencies. To limit your investigation to research studies and osteopathy, you will need to use the advanced search options. First, go to **http://chid.nih.gov/index.html**. From there, select the "Detailed Search" option (or go directly to that page with the following hyperlink: **http://chid.nih.gov/detail/detail.html**). The trick in extracting studies is found in the drop boxes at the bottom of the search page where "You may refine your search by." Select the dates and language you prefer, and the format option "Journal Article." At the top of the search form, select the number of records you would like to see (we recommend 100) and check the box to display "whole records." We recommend that you type "osteopathy" (or synonyms) into the "For these words:" box. Consider using the option "anywhere in record" to make your search as broad as possible. If you want to limit the search to only a particular field, such as the title of the journal, then select this option in the "Search in these fields" drop box. The following is what you can expect from this type of search:

- **Paradox of Osteopathy**

    Source: New England Journal of Medicine. 341(19): 1465-1468. November 4, 1999.

    Summary: This journal article reviews the history of **osteopathy** and its changing relationship with allopathic medicine. **Osteopathy** was originally created in the late 19th century as an alternative to the existing system of medicine. Chiropractic was established about the same time. Both disciplines, initially parts of a pluralistic medical system, have taken different paths over the course of the 20th century. Chiropractors generally have remained focused on spinal manipulation for a limited set of conditions. Osteopaths, on the other hand, have moved closer to allopathy and tend to rely less on osteopathic manipulation as the primary treatment modality. In this author's opinion, however, the future of osteopathic medicine depends on its ability to define itself as distinct from and yet still equivalent to allopathic medicine. The article has 19 references.

Federally Funded Research on Osteopathy

The U.S. Government supports a variety of research studies relating to osteopathy. These studies are tracked by the Office of Extramural Research at the National Institutes of Health.[2] CRISP (Computerized Retrieval of Information on Scientific Projects) is a searchable database of federally funded biomedical research projects conducted at universities, hospitals, and other institutions.

Search the CRISP Web site at **http://crisp.cit.nih.gov/crisp/crisp_query.generate_screen**. You will have the option to perform targeted searches by various criteria, including geography, date, and topics related to osteopathy.

For most of the studies, the agencies reporting into CRISP provide summaries or abstracts. As opposed to clinical trial research using patients, many federally funded studies use animals or simulated models to explore osteopathy. The following is typical of the type of information found when searching the CRISP database for osteopathy:

- **Project Title: HARVARD MENTORED CLINICAL SCIENTIST DEVELOPMENT PROGRAM**

  Principal Investigator & Institution: Lipsitz, Lewis A.; Professor of Medicine; Divison on Aging; Harvard University (Medical School) Medical School Campus Boston, Ma 02115

  Timing: Fiscal Year 2002; Project Start 01-AUG-1985; Project End 30-JUN-2004

  Summary: This revised competing renewal proposal seeks support to continue a highly successful, NIA-funded Mentored Clinical Scientist Development Program Award. The program represents a major, multidisciplinary and interdepartmental collaboration among the medical school, school of public health, as well as the affiliated institutions in the Longwood Medical Area and around Boston. We have increased our efforts at recruiting candidates widely, including those who are members of under-represented minorities in aging research, and those who are from other medical schools including schools of **osteopathy**. We have provided information on eight superb prospective trainee candidates of which five are women, three are African American, one is Hispanic, and one is a doctor of **osteopathy** working with underserved elderly (including Native Americans) in rural Maine. Many of these candidates are interested in pursuing research in public and social medicine, especially the care of minority elderly in the underserved, inner-city and underserved rural communities of America. The proposed Program is designed to support and enhance research experience in several interrelated gerontologic disciplines. Six specific areas will be emphasized. These are (1) cardiovascular disease, (2) cell proliferation disorders, (3) neurodegenerative disease and dementia, (4) endocrine/renal dysfunction, (5) geriatric syndromes, and (6) public health. More than 50 experienced, well-funded faculty scientists (20 of whom are women), many of whom are established gerontologic investigators, will serve as potential primary or secondary mentors for the clinician scientist trainees. A dual

---

[2] Healthcare projects are funded by the National Institutes of Health (NIH), Substance Abuse and Mental Health Services (SAMHSA), Health Resources and Services Administration (HRSA), Food and Drug Administration (FDA), Centers for Disease Control and Prevention (CDCP), Agency for Healthcare Research and Quality (AHRQ), and Office of Assistant Secretary of Health (OASH).

mentoring system has been implemented to ensure ongoing exposure to gerontologic/geriatric expertise and orientation. Ultimately, we plan to develop the trainees into clinician investigators who can facilitate the translation of important research findings into improved care for all older Americans.

Website: http://crisp.cit.nih.gov/crisp/Crisp_Query.Generate_Screen

- **Project Title: OSTEOPATHIC MANIPULATIVE MEDICINE**

Principal Investigator & Institution: Stoll, Scott T.; Chairman and Associate Professor; Manipulative Medicine; University of North Texas Hlth Sci Ctr Fort Worth, Tx 761072699

Timing: Fiscal Year 2002; Project Start 28-SEP-2000; Project End 31-JUL-2005

Summary: (Applicant's Abstract): The Physical Medicine Institute in conjunction with the Department of Osteopathic Manipulative Medicine (OMM) formalized a Predoctoral Research Fellowship in OMM at the University of North Texas Health Science Center in 1998 as an extension of a Predoctoral Teaching Fellowship in OMM founded 1985. This program was designed to develop successful researchers in complementary & alternative medicine (CAM), specifically OMM. It collaborates with the School of Public Health, Graduate School of Biomedical Sciences, & various departments of Clinical Medicine; & is coordinating efforts to offer predoctoral fellows the combined D.O./M.P.H. degree through enrollment in a variety of research & CAM related courses. We propose to enhance the administrative, curricular, mentoring, & funding structures of the current research program. Development is targeted at: (1) curriculum expansion with courses on hypothesis building; biostatistics; epidemiology; clinical trial design; research methods; responsible conduct; ethical & regulatory issues in research, (2) development of new CAM-focused courses; (3) program extension to attract a wider audience including faculty, pre- and post- doctoral fellows, & allied health professionals; (4) establishment of annual CAM research conferences; (5) development of Continuing Medical Education courses in CAM; (6) formalization of various degree tracks; & (7) use of computer technologies for curricular advancement. Research fellows will acquire the skills necessary to successfully develop basic science & clinical research projects, attain funding, implement studies & publish quality research in CAM with the opportunity to advance toward various degrees in combination with or addition to their Doctor of **Osteopathy** degree. Fellows, at present, are competitively selected from a diverse multicultural pool of osteopathic medical students from the UNTHSC. This evolving predoctoral fellowship program has a successful track record of graduating accomplished clinical researchers, educators & administrators in OMM. This expanded & improved program will continue to develop future leaders and researchers capable of successful and competitive clinical & basic science research in CAM.

Website: http://crisp.cit.nih.gov/crisp/Crisp_Query.Generate_Screen

- **Project Title: SUPPORT FOR OSTEOPATHIC RESEARCH CONFERENCE**

Principal Investigator & Institution: Rose, Richard C.; American Osteopathic Association 142 E Ontario St Chicago, Il 60611

Timing: Fiscal Year 2003; Project Start 15-SEP-2003; Project End 31-DEC-2003

Summary: (provided by applicant): The goal is to hold a research conference sponsored by the American Osteopathic Association in New Orleans, LA on October 12-15, 2003. The title is "Evidence-Base for the use of Osteopathic Manipulative Medicine in Clinical Practice". Twelve speakers have been selected who agree to present new and original research data regarding the use of osteopathic manipulative medicine (OMM) in clinical practice. In that each topic is a specific use of OMM, and that OMM is considered a form of CAM, the program should be of interest to NCCAM Also, because many of the medical conditions to be featured in the program are musculoskeletal, the program should be of interest to NIAMS. Finally, because the medical conditions are more prevalent in the elderly, the conference may be of interest to NIA. The didactic session format allows for four 30-40 minute presentations on each of three mornings. This promotes interaction in an intimate setting of investigators who have overlapping clinical interests. This is a fertile setting for generating additional collaboration and research plans. We are arranging joint sponsorship of one-third of the Conference with the American Academy of **Osteopathy.** Members of the Academy are particularly interested in manipulative medicine in the treatment of musculoskeletal disorders. A second component of the Conference that features original research is the poster session. We expect approximately 100 abstracts will be submitted to the AOA, reviewed by the Council on Research Grants and that most will be found to contain original research data as required for acceptance. Publication in the Journal of the American Osteopathic Association and presentation at the Conference in poster format will follow. The poster session includes a student research prize competition.

Website: http://crisp.cit.nih.gov/crisp/Crisp_Query.Generate_Screen

E-Journals: PubMed Central[3]

PubMed Central (PMC) is a digital archive of life sciences journal literature developed and managed by the National Center for Biotechnology Information (NCBI) at the U.S. National Library of Medicine (NLM).[4] Access to this growing archive of e-journals is free and unrestricted.[5] To search, go to **http://www.ncbi.nlm.nih.gov/entrez/query.fcgi?db=Pmc**, and type "osteopathy" (or synonyms) into the search box. This search gives you access to full-text articles. The following is a sample of items found for osteopathy in the PubMed Central database:

- **Craniomandibular osteopathy in a bullmastiff.** by Huchkowsky SL.; 2002 Nov; http://www.pubmedcentral.gov/articlerender.fcgi?tool=pmcentrez&artid=339767

The National Library of Medicine: PubMed

One of the quickest and most comprehensive ways to find academic studies in both English and other languages is to use PubMed, maintained by the National Library of Medicine.[6] The advantage of PubMed over previously mentioned sources is that it covers a greater number of domestic and foreign references. It is also free to use. If the publisher has a Web

---

[3] Adapted from the National Library of Medicine: **http://www.pubmedcentral.nih.gov/about/intro.html**.

[4] With PubMed Central, NCBI is taking the lead in preservation and maintenance of open access to electronic literature, just as NLM has done for decades with printed biomedical literature. PubMed Central aims to become a world-class library of the digital age.

[5] The value of PubMed Central, in addition to its role as an archive, lies in the availability of data from diverse sources stored in a common format in a single repository. Many journals already have online publishing operations, and there is a growing tendency to publish material online only, to the exclusion of print.

[6] PubMed was developed by the National Center for Biotechnology Information (NCBI) at the National Library of Medicine (NLM) at the National Institutes of Health (NIH). The PubMed database was developed in conjunction with publishers of biomedical literature as a search tool for accessing literature citations and linking to full-text journal articles at Web sites of participating publishers. Publishers that participate in PubMed supply NLM with their citations electronically prior to or at the time of publication.

site that offers full text of its journals, PubMed will provide links to that site, as well as to sites offering other related data. User registration, a subscription fee, or some other type of fee may be required to access the full text of articles in some journals.

To generate your own bibliography of studies dealing with osteopathy, simply go to the PubMed Web site at **http://www.ncbi.nlm.nih.gov/pubmed**. Type "osteopathy" (or synonyms) into the search box, and click "Go." The following is the type of output you can expect from PubMed for osteopathy (hyperlinks lead to article summaries):

- **"Traditional osteopathy": an oxymoron?**
  Author(s): Findlay T.
  Source: J Am Osteopath Assoc. 2000 September; 100(9): 545. No Abstract Available.
  http://www.ncbi.nlm.nih.gov/entrez/query.fcgi?cmd=Retrieve&db=pubmed&dopt=Abstract&list_uids=11057071

- **ABC of complementary medicine. The manipulative therapies: osteopathy and chiropractic.**
  Author(s): Vickers A, Zollman C.
  Source: Bmj (Clinical Research Ed.). 1999 October 30; 319(7218): 1176-9. Review.
  http://www.ncbi.nlm.nih.gov/entrez/query.fcgi?cmd=Retrieve&db=pubmed&dopt=Abstract&list_uids=10541511

- **Alkaline phosphatase bone isoenzyme activity in serum in various degrees of micromorphometrically assessed renal osteopathy.**
  Author(s): Siede WH, Seiffert UB, Bundschuh F, Malluche HH, Schoeppe W.
  Source: Clinical Nephrology. 1980 June; 13(6): 277-81.
  http://www.ncbi.nlm.nih.gov/entrez/query.fcgi?cmd=Retrieve&db=pubmed&dopt=Abstract&list_uids=7408246

- **Aluminum osteopathy.**
  Author(s): Cournot-Witmer G.
  Source: Contrib Nephrol. 1984; 38: 59-64. No Abstract Available.
  http://www.ncbi.nlm.nih.gov/entrez/query.fcgi?cmd=Retrieve&db=pubmed&dopt=Abstract&list_uids=6713901

- **Andrew Taylor Still, M.D.: founder of osteopathy.**
  Author(s): Burns SB, Burns JL.
  Source: Journal of Alternative and Complementary Medicine (New York, N.Y.). 1997 Fall; 3(3): 213-4. Erratum In: J Altern Complement Med 1997 Winter; 3(4): 321.
  http://www.ncbi.nlm.nih.gov/entrez/query.fcgi?cmd=Retrieve&db=pubmed&dopt=Abstract&list_uids=9430324

- **Bone scintigraphy and radiography in the early recognition of diabetic osteopathy.**
  Author(s): Tawn DJ, O'Hare JP, O'Brien IA, Watt I, Dieppe PA, Corrall RJ.
  Source: The British Journal of Radiology. 1988 April; 61(724): 273-9.
  http://www.ncbi.nlm.nih.gov/entrez/query.fcgi?cmd=Retrieve&db=pubmed&dopt=Abstract&list_uids=3370410

- **Cadmium-induced osteopathy: clinical and autopsy findings of four patients.**
  Author(s): Takebayashi S, Harada T, Kamura S, Satoh T, Segawa M, Yajima K.
  Source: Appl Pathol. 1987; 5(3): 190-7.
  http://www.ncbi.nlm.nih.gov/entrez/query.fcgi?cmd=Retrieve&db=pubmed&dopt=Abstract&list_uids=3620212

- **Calcium metabolism and osteopathy in diabetes mellitus.**
  Author(s): Shao AH, Wang FG, Hu YF, Zhang LM.
  Source: Contrib Nephrol. 1991; 90: 212-6.
  http://www.ncbi.nlm.nih.gov/entrez/query.fcgi?cmd=Retrieve&db=pubmed&dopt=Abstract&list_uids=1959349

- **Canine distemper virus transcripts detected in the bone cells of dogs with metaphyseal osteopathy.**
  Author(s): Mee AP, Gordon MT, May C, Bennett D, Anderson DC, Sharpe PT.
  Source: Bone. 1993; 14(1): 59-67.
  http://www.ncbi.nlm.nih.gov/entrez/query.fcgi?cmd=Retrieve&db=pubmed&dopt=Abstract&list_uids=8443004

- **c-kit mutation and osteopetrosis-like osteopathy in a patient with systemic mast cell disease.**
  Author(s): Reinacher-Schick A, Petrasch S, Longley BJ, Teschendorf C, Graeven U, Schmiegel W.
  Source: Annals of Hematology. 1998 September; 77(3): 131-4.
  http://www.ncbi.nlm.nih.gov/entrez/query.fcgi?cmd=Retrieve&db=pubmed&dopt=Abstract&list_uids=9797083

- **Clinical images: aluminum-modified renal osteopathy.**
  Author(s): Buttgereit F, Loreck D, Burmester GR, Abendroth K.
  Source: Arthritis and Rheumatism. 1997 September; 40(9): 1724.
  http://www.ncbi.nlm.nih.gov/entrez/query.fcgi?cmd=Retrieve&db=pubmed&dopt=Abstract&list_uids=9324031

- **Clinical problems of renal osteopathy in patients on hemofiltration.**
  Author(s): Schulz W, Baier E, Humpfner A, Delling G.
  Source: Contrib Nephrol. 1982; 32: 86-91. No Abstract Available.
  http://www.ncbi.nlm.nih.gov/entrez/query.fcgi?cmd=Retrieve&db=pubmed&dopt=Abstract&list_uids=7128166

- **Complementary medicine. Osteopathy.**
  Author(s): Trevelyan J.
  Source: Nurs Times. 1993 August 25-31; 89(34): 46-8. No Abstract Available.
  http://www.ncbi.nlm.nih.gov/entrez/query.fcgi?cmd=Retrieve&db=pubmed&dopt=Abstract&list_uids=8139945

- **Computer evaluation to the x-ray densitometry method for the diagnosis of calcipenic osteopathy.**
  Author(s): Bojtor I, Illes A, Horvath F, Hollo I.
  Source: Fortschr Geb Rontgenstr Nuklearmed. 1972 December; 117(6): 720-4. No Abstract Available.
  http://www.ncbi.nlm.nih.gov/entrez/query.fcgi?cmd=Retrieve&db=pubmed&dopt=Abstract&list_uids=4346207

- **Cranial osteopathy and its role in disorders of the temporomandibular joint.**
  Author(s): Frymann VM.
  Source: Dent Clin North Am. 1983 July; 27(3): 595-611. No Abstract Available.
  http://www.ncbi.nlm.nih.gov/entrez/query.fcgi?cmd=Retrieve&db=pubmed&dopt=Abstract&list_uids=6578968

- **Cranial osteopathy.**
  Author(s): Holmes P.
  Source: Nurs Times. 1991 May 29-June 4; 87(22): 36-8. No Abstract Available.
  http://www.ncbi.nlm.nih.gov/entrez/query.fcgi?cmd=Retrieve&db=pubmed&dopt=Abstract&list_uids=2041821

- **Cranial osteopathy.**
  Author(s): Bowden R.
  Source: Australas Nurses J. 1983 March; 12(1): 3-5. No Abstract Available.
  http://www.ncbi.nlm.nih.gov/entrez/query.fcgi?cmd=Retrieve&db=pubmed&dopt=Abstract&list_uids=6555031

- **Dental equilibration and osteopathy.**
  Author(s): Magoun HI Sr.
  Source: J Am Osteopath Assoc. 1975 June; 74(10): 981-91. No Abstract Available.
  http://www.ncbi.nlm.nih.gov/entrez/query.fcgi?cmd=Retrieve&db=pubmed&dopt=Abstract&list_uids=1040000

- **Diabetes mellitus with osteopathy and Charcot's arthropathy.**
  Author(s): Rosenberg JN.
  Source: Proc R Soc Med. 1976 September; 69(9): 705. No Abstract Available.
  http://www.ncbi.nlm.nih.gov/entrez/query.fcgi?cmd=Retrieve&db=pubmed&dopt=Abstract&list_uids=981276

- **Diabetic osteopathy of the foot and ankle.**
  Author(s): Finby N, Kraft E, Spyropoulos E.
  Source: American Family Physician. 1976 September; 14(3): 90-5.
  http://www.ncbi.nlm.nih.gov/entrez/query.fcgi?cmd=Retrieve&db=pubmed&dopt=Abstract&list_uids=961565

- **Diabetic osteopathy.**
  Author(s): Griffiths HJ.
  Source: Orthopedics. 1985 March; 8(3): 398, 401-6.
  http://www.ncbi.nlm.nih.gov/entrez/query.fcgi?cmd=Retrieve&db=pubmed&dopt=Abstract&list_uids=4094983

- **Diabetic osteopathy: report of a relentlessly progressive case, with clinico-pathologic correlations.**
  Author(s): Shagan BP, Friedman SA, Allesandri R.
  Source: Journal of the American Geriatrics Society. 1973 December; 21(12): 561-5.
  http://www.ncbi.nlm.nih.gov/entrez/query.fcgi?cmd=Retrieve&db=pubmed&dopt=Abstract&list_uids=4749427

- **Distribution of health services in Missouri: I. Doctors of medicine and osteopathy.**
  Author(s): Baker AS, Bishop FM, Hassinger EW, Hobbs DJ.
  Source: Mo Med. 1967 October; 64(10): 856-62. No Abstract Available.
  http://www.ncbi.nlm.nih.gov/entrez/query.fcgi?cmd=Retrieve&db=pubmed&dopt=Abstract&list_uids=6072876

- **Effect of parathyroidectomy on thyrotropic and lactotropic function in patients with renal osteopathy.**
  Author(s): Zofkova I, Sotornik I.
  Source: Nephron. 1995; 71(3): 284-90.
  http://www.ncbi.nlm.nih.gov/entrez/query.fcgi?cmd=Retrieve&db=pubmed&dopt=Abstract&list_uids=8569976

- **Hypocalcemia and osteopathy in mice with kidney-specific megalin gene defect.**
  Author(s): Leheste JR, Melsen F, Wellner M, Jansen P, Schlichting U, Renner-Muller I, Andreassen TT, Wolf E, Bachmann S, Nykjaer A, Willnow TE.
  Source: The Faseb Journal : Official Publication of the Federation of American Societies for Experimental Biology. 2003 February; 17(2): 247-9. Epub 2002 December 03.
  http://www.ncbi.nlm.nih.gov/entrez/query.fcgi?cmd=Retrieve&db=pubmed&dopt=Abstract&list_uids=12475886

- **Infantile cortical hyperostosis (Caffey-Silverman syndrome). Animal model: craniomandibular osteopathy in the canine.**
  Author(s): Thornburg LP.
  Source: American Journal of Pathology. 1979 May; 95(2): 575-8.
  http://www.ncbi.nlm.nih.gov/entrez/query.fcgi?cmd=Retrieve&db=pubmed&dopt=Abstract&list_uids=377993

- **Integrating cranial osteopathy with gnathologic orthopedics.**
  Author(s): Kennedy JM.
  Source: J Am Acad Gnathol Orthop. 1998 September; 15(3): 4-9. No Abstract Available.
  http://www.ncbi.nlm.nih.gov/entrez/query.fcgi?cmd=Retrieve&db=pubmed&dopt=Abstract&list_uids=10597141

- **Integrating cranial osteopathy with gnathologic orthopedics.**
  Author(s): Kennedy JM.
  Source: J Am Acad Gnathol Orthop. 1998 June; 15(2): 4-7 Contd. No Abstract Available.
  http://www.ncbi.nlm.nih.gov/entrez/query.fcgi?cmd=Retrieve&db=pubmed&dopt=Abstract&list_uids=10596640

- **Introducing the cranial approach in osteopathy and the treatment of infants and mothers.**
  Author(s): Sullivan C.
  Source: Complementary Therapies in Nursing & Midwifery. 1997 June; 3(3): 72-6. Review.
  http://www.ncbi.nlm.nih.gov/entrez/query.fcgi?cmd=Retrieve&db=pubmed&dopt=Abstract&list_uids=9439253

- **Investigations of bone turnover in renal osteopathy.**
  Author(s): Muller A, Stein G, Lehmann G, Hein G.
  Source: European Journal of Medical Research. 1999 February 25; 4(2): 78-84.
  http://www.ncbi.nlm.nih.gov/entrez/query.fcgi?cmd=Retrieve&db=pubmed&dopt=Abstract&list_uids=10066644

- **Iron as a possible aggravating factor for osteopathy in itai-itai disease, a disease associated with chronic cadmium intoxication.**
  Author(s): Noda M, Yasuda M, Kitagawa M.
  Source: Journal of Bone and Mineral Research : the Official Journal of the American Society for Bone and Mineral Research. 1991 March; 6(3): 245-55.
  http://www.ncbi.nlm.nih.gov/entrez/query.fcgi?cmd=Retrieve&db=pubmed&dopt=Abstract&list_uids=2035351

- **Is methotrexate osteopathy a form of bone idiosyncrasy?**
  Author(s): Rozin AP.
  Source: Annals of the Rheumatic Diseases. 2003 November; 62(11): 1123; Author Reply 1124.
  http://www.ncbi.nlm.nih.gov/entrez/query.fcgi?cmd=Retrieve&db=pubmed&dopt=Abstract&list_uids=14583585

- **Is there a psoriatic osteopathy? -- the activity of bone resorption in psoriatics is related to inflammatory joint process.**
  Author(s): Hein G, Schmidt F, Barta U, Muller A.
  Source: European Journal of Medical Research. 1999 May 26; 4(5): 187-92.
  http://www.ncbi.nlm.nih.gov/entrez/query.fcgi?cmd=Retrieve&db=pubmed&dopt=Abstract&list_uids=10336408

- **Letter: Striated osteopathy in focal dermal hypoplasia.**
  Author(s): Larregue M, Duterque M.
  Source: Archives of Dermatology. 1975 October; 111(10): 1365.
  http://www.ncbi.nlm.nih.gov/entrez/query.fcgi?cmd=Retrieve&db=pubmed&dopt=Abstract&list_uids=1190805

- **Long-term CaCO3 treatment of chronic hemodialysis patients: an attempt to prevent aluminum osteopathy.**
  Author(s): Matsubara M, Unagami H, Totsune K, Sato H, Kikuta Y, Ogawa M, Saito T, Yoshinaga K.
  Source: Asaio Trans. 1988 July-September; 34(3): 168-71.
  http://www.ncbi.nlm.nih.gov/entrez/query.fcgi?cmd=Retrieve&db=pubmed&dopt=Abstract&list_uids=3196505

- **Low dose methotrexate osteopathy in a patient with polyarticular juvenile idiopathic arthritis.**
  Author(s): Quinn MA, Green MJ, Gough AK.
  Source: Annals of the Rheumatic Diseases. 2003 November; 62(11): 1123-4; Author Reply 1124.
  http://www.ncbi.nlm.nih.gov/entrez/query.fcgi?cmd=Retrieve&db=pubmed&dopt=Abstract&list_uids=14583584

- **Low dose methotrexate osteopathy in a patient with polyarticular juvenile idiopathic arthritis.**
  Author(s): Rudler M, Pouchot J, Paycha F, Gentelle S, Grasland A, Vinceneux P.
  Source: Annals of the Rheumatic Diseases. 2003 June; 62(6): 588-9.
  http://www.ncbi.nlm.nih.gov/entrez/query.fcgi?cmd=Retrieve&db=pubmed&dopt=Abstract&list_uids=12759303

- **Managing back pain in general practice--is osteopathy the new paradigm?**
  Author(s): Williams N.
  Source: The British Journal of General Practice : the Journal of the Royal College of General Practitioners. 1997 October; 47(423): 653-5. Review.
  http://www.ncbi.nlm.nih.gov/entrez/query.fcgi?cmd=Retrieve&db=pubmed&dopt=Abstract&list_uids=9474832

- **Manipulation, osteopathy, and back pain.**
  Author(s): Dove CI.
  Source: Lancet. 1979 June 23; 1(8130): 1350.
  http://www.ncbi.nlm.nih.gov/entrez/query.fcgi?cmd=Retrieve&db=pubmed&dopt=Abstract&list_uids=87812

- **Methotrexate (MTX) inhibits osteoblastic differentiation in vitro: possible mechanism of MTX osteopathy.**
  Author(s): Uehara R, Suzuki Y, Ichikawa Y.
  Source: The Journal of Rheumatology. 2001 February; 28(2): 251-6.
  http://www.ncbi.nlm.nih.gov/entrez/query.fcgi?cmd=Retrieve&db=pubmed&dopt=Abstract&list_uids=11246658

- **Methotrexate osteopathy demonstrated by Technetium-99m HDP bone scintigraphy.**
  Author(s): Stevens H, Jacobs JW, Van Rijk PP, De Klerk JM.
  Source: Clinical Nuclear Medicine. 2001 May; 26(5): 389-91.
  http://www.ncbi.nlm.nih.gov/entrez/query.fcgi?cmd=Retrieve&db=pubmed&dopt=Abstract&list_uids=11317015

- **Methotrexate osteopathy in infants with tumors of the central nervous system.**
  Author(s): Meister B, Gassner I, Streif W, Dengg K, Fink FM.
  Source: Medical and Pediatric Oncology. 1994; 23(6): 493-6.
  http://www.ncbi.nlm.nih.gov/entrez/query.fcgi?cmd=Retrieve&db=pubmed&dopt=Abstract&list_uids=7935176

- **Methotrexate osteopathy in long-term, low-dose methotrexate treatment for psoriasis and rheumatoid arthritis.**
  Author(s): Zonneveld IM, Bakker WK, Dijkstra PF, Bos JD, van Soesbergen RM, Dinant HJ.
  Source: Archives of Dermatology. 1996 February; 132(2): 184-7.
  http://www.ncbi.nlm.nih.gov/entrez/query.fcgi?cmd=Retrieve&db=pubmed&dopt=Abstract&list_uids=8629827

- **Methotrexate osteopathy in patients with osteosarcoma.**
  Author(s): Ecklund K, Laor T, Goorin AM, Connolly LP, Jaramillo D.
  Source: Radiology. 1997 February; 202(2): 543-7.
  http://www.ncbi.nlm.nih.gov/entrez/query.fcgi?cmd=Retrieve&db=pubmed&dopt=Abstract&list_uids=9015088

- **Methotrexate osteopathy in rheumatic disease.**
  Author(s): Preston SJ, Diamond T, Scott A, Laurent MR.
  Source: Annals of the Rheumatic Diseases. 1993 August; 52(8): 582-5.
  http://www.ncbi.nlm.nih.gov/entrez/query.fcgi?cmd=Retrieve&db=pubmed&dopt=Abstract&list_uids=8215620

- **Methotrexate osteopathy, does it exist?**
  Author(s): Maenaut K, Westhovens R, Dequeker J.
  Source: The Journal of Rheumatology. 1996 December; 23(12): 2156-9.
  http://www.ncbi.nlm.nih.gov/entrez/query.fcgi?cmd=Retrieve&db=pubmed&dopt=Abstract&list_uids=8970056

- **Methotrexate osteopathy.**
  Author(s): Rooney P.
  Source: The Journal of Rheumatology. 1997 October; 24(10): 2051.
  http://www.ncbi.nlm.nih.gov/entrez/query.fcgi?cmd=Retrieve&db=pubmed&dopt=Abstract&list_uids=9330955

- **Methotrexate osteopathy.**
  Author(s): Schwartz AM, Leonidas JC.
  Source: Skeletal Radiology. 1984; 11(1): 13-6.
  http://www.ncbi.nlm.nih.gov/entrez/query.fcgi?cmd=Retrieve&db=pubmed&dopt=Abstract&list_uids=6424236

- **Midwifery. Osteopathy during pregnancy.**
  Author(s): Montague K.
  Source: Nurs Mirror. 1985 July 31; 161(5): 26-8. No Abstract Available.
  http://www.ncbi.nlm.nih.gov/entrez/query.fcgi?cmd=Retrieve&db=pubmed&dopt=Abstract&list_uids=3161004

- **Morphometry of bone. Are parameters from the iliac crest reliable indicators of renal-insufficiency osteopathy?**
  Author(s): Oberholzer M, Remagen W, Orfei R, Ehrsam RE, Heitz PU.
  Source: Anal Quant Cytol Histol. 1986 September; 8(3): 250-4.
  http://www.ncbi.nlm.nih.gov/entrez/query.fcgi?cmd=Retrieve&db=pubmed&dopt=Abstract&list_uids=3778618

- **Non-aluminic adynamic bone disease in non-dialyzed uremic patients: a new type of osteopathy due to overtreatment?**
  Author(s): Cohen-Solal ME, Sebert JL, Boudailliez B, Westeel PF, Moriniere PH, Marie A, Garabedian M, Fournier A.
  Source: Bone. 1992; 13(1): 1-5.
  http://www.ncbi.nlm.nih.gov/entrez/query.fcgi?cmd=Retrieve&db=pubmed&dopt=Abstract&list_uids=1581102

- **Nonosteomalacic osteopathy associated with chronic hypophosphatemia.**
  Author(s): de Vernejoul MC, Marie P, Kuntz D, Gueris J, Miravet L, Ryckewaert A.
  Source: Calcified Tissue International. 1982 May; 34(3): 219-23.
  http://www.ncbi.nlm.nih.gov/entrez/query.fcgi?cmd=Retrieve&db=pubmed&dopt=Abstract&list_uids=6809281

- **On diabetic osteopathy: a radiographic study of 21 patients.**
  Author(s): Whitehouse FW, Weckstein M.
  Source: Diabetes Care. 1978 September-October; 1(5): 303-4.
  http://www.ncbi.nlm.nih.gov/entrez/query.fcgi?cmd=Retrieve&db=pubmed&dopt=Abstract&list_uids=720184

- **Osteoclastogenesis and osteoclast activation in dialysis-related amyloid osteopathy.**
  Author(s): Kazama JJ, Maruyama H, Gejyo F.
  Source: American Journal of Kidney Diseases : the Official Journal of the National Kidney Foundation. 2001 October; 38(4 Suppl 1): S156-60. Review.
  http://www.ncbi.nlm.nih.gov/entrez/query.fcgi?cmd=Retrieve&db=pubmed&dopt=Abstract&list_uids=11576944

- **Osteomyelitis of both femora in a patient on maintenance hemodialysis with severe uremic osteopathy.**
  Author(s): Krempien B, Ritz E.
  Source: Virchows Arch a Pathol Pathol Anat. 1972; 356(2): 119-26. No Abstract Available.
  http://www.ncbi.nlm.nih.gov/entrez/query.fcgi?cmd=Retrieve&db=pubmed&dopt=Abstract&list_uids=4626947

- **Osteopathy an independent system co-extensive with the science and art of healing. 1901.**
  Author(s): Littlejohn JM.
  Source: J Am Osteopath Assoc. 2000 January; 100(1): 14-26. No Abstract Available.
  http://www.ncbi.nlm.nih.gov/entrez/query.fcgi?cmd=Retrieve&db=pubmed&dopt=Abstract&list_uids=10693313

- **Osteopathy and back pain.**
  Author(s): Ruddick D.
  Source: Nursing (Lond). 1979 June; (3): 150-2. No Abstract Available.
  http://www.ncbi.nlm.nih.gov/entrez/query.fcgi?cmd=Retrieve&db=pubmed&dopt=Abstract&list_uids=161363

- **Osteopathy and insanity. 1917.**
  Author(s): Gerdine LV.
  Source: J Am Osteopath Assoc. 2000 August; 100(8): 499-500. No Abstract Available.
  http://www.ncbi.nlm.nih.gov/entrez/query.fcgi?cmd=Retrieve&db=pubmed&dopt=Abstract&list_uids=10979257

- **Osteopathy due to methotrexate.**
  Author(s): Koller A, Fill H, Kurz R, Riccabona G, Haas H.
  Source: Osterr Kneipp Mag. 1976 September 13; 3(3): 63-9.
  http://www.ncbi.nlm.nih.gov/entrez/query.fcgi?cmd=Retrieve&db=pubmed&dopt=Abstract&list_uids=1069959

- **Osteopathy in back trouble.**
  Author(s): Burton AK.
  Source: British Medical Journal (Clinical Research Ed.). 1986 December 6; 293(6560): 1482-3.
  http://www.ncbi.nlm.nih.gov/entrez/query.fcgi?cmd=Retrieve&db=pubmed&dopt=Abstract&list_uids=2948610

- **Osteopathy in general practice.**
  Author(s): Burns K, Lyttelton L.
  Source: The British Journal of General Practice : the Journal of the Royal College of General Practitioners. 1994 February; 44(379): 93.
  http://www.ncbi.nlm.nih.gov/entrez/query.fcgi?cmd=Retrieve&db=pubmed&dopt=Abstract&list_uids=8179955

- **Osteopathy in general practice.**
  Author(s): Griffin GA.
  Source: Proc R Soc Med. 1973 May; 66(5): 423-5. No Abstract Available.
  http://www.ncbi.nlm.nih.gov/entrez/query.fcgi?cmd=Retrieve&db=pubmed&dopt=Abstract&list_uids=4268526

- **Osteopathy in hyperthyroidism--a study of 47 calcium kinetics and quantitative histology of bone.**
  Author(s): Montz R, Hehrmann R, Langbein H, Schneider C, Haug HP, Delling G.
  Source: Acta Endocrinol Suppl (Copenh). 1973; 173: 146. No Abstract Available.
  http://www.ncbi.nlm.nih.gov/entrez/query.fcgi?cmd=Retrieve&db=pubmed&dopt=Abstract&list_uids=4542078

- **Osteopathy in its early adulthood, 1945-1955.**
  Author(s): Patterson MM.
  Source: J Am Osteopath Assoc. 2001 January; 101(1): 33. No Abstract Available.
  http://www.ncbi.nlm.nih.gov/entrez/query.fcgi?cmd=Retrieve&db=pubmed&dopt=Abstract&list_uids=11234219

- **Osteopathy in maintenance hemodialysis.**
  Author(s): Krempien B, Ritz E, Beck U, Keilbach H.
  Source: Virchows Arch a Pathol Pathol Anat. 1972; 357(4): 257-74. No Abstract Available.
  http://www.ncbi.nlm.nih.gov/entrez/query.fcgi?cmd=Retrieve&db=pubmed&dopt=Abstract&list_uids=4629286

- **Osteopathy in pregnancy and childbirth. Interview by Jenny Green.**
  Author(s): Sandler S, Korth S.
  Source: Pract Midwife. 2000 July-August; 3(7): 38-43. No Abstract Available.
  http://www.ncbi.nlm.nih.gov/entrez/query.fcgi?cmd=Retrieve&db=pubmed&dopt=A
  bstract&list_uids=12026438

- **Osteopathy in the cranial field: uncovering challenges and potential applications.**
  Author(s): King HH.
  Source: J Am Osteopath Assoc. 2002 July; 102(7): 367-9. No Abstract Available.
  http://www.ncbi.nlm.nih.gov/entrez/query.fcgi?cmd=Retrieve&db=pubmed&dopt=A
  bstract&list_uids=12138950

- **Osteopathy vs chiropractic.**
  Author(s): Friedman H.
  Source: The Journal of Family Practice. 1993 September; 37(3): 221-2.
  http://www.ncbi.nlm.nih.gov/entrez/query.fcgi?cmd=Retrieve&db=pubmed&dopt=A
  bstract&list_uids=8409868

- **Osteopathy, chiropractic, and spinal manipulation.**
  Author(s): Patmas MA.
  Source: Annals of Internal Medicine. 1993 April 15; 118(8): 652; Author Reply 652-3.
  http://www.ncbi.nlm.nih.gov/entrez/query.fcgi?cmd=Retrieve&db=pubmed&dopt=A
  bstract&list_uids=8452341

- **Osteopathy, chiropractic, and spinal manipulation.**
  Author(s): Plaugher G.
  Source: Annals of Internal Medicine. 1993 April 15; 118(8): 651; Author Reply 652-3.
  http://www.ncbi.nlm.nih.gov/entrez/query.fcgi?cmd=Retrieve&db=pubmed&dopt=A
  bstract&list_uids=8452339

- **Osteopathy, chiropractic, and spinal manipulation.**
  Author(s): Abend DS.
  Source: Annals of Internal Medicine. 1993 April 15; 118(8): 651; Author Reply 652-3.
  http://www.ncbi.nlm.nih.gov/entrez/query.fcgi?cmd=Retrieve&db=pubmed&dopt=A
  bstract&list_uids=8318092

- **Osteopathy.**
  Author(s): Wilkinson MJ.
  Source: The British Journal of General Practice : the Journal of the Royal College of
  General Practitioners. 1993 June; 43(371): 261-2.
  http://www.ncbi.nlm.nih.gov/entrez/query.fcgi?cmd=Retrieve&db=pubmed&dopt=A
  bstract&list_uids=8373654

- **Osteopathy.**
  Author(s): MacDonald RS, Peters D.
  Source: The Practitioner. 1986 December; 230(1422): 1073-6.
  http://www.ncbi.nlm.nih.gov/entrez/query.fcgi?cmd=Retrieve&db=pubmed&dopt=A
  bstract&list_uids=3671312

- **Osteopathy.**
  Author(s): Dove CI.
  Source: Midwife Health Visit Community Nurse. 1983 September; 19(9): 358-65. No Abstract Available.
  http://www.ncbi.nlm.nih.gov/entrez/query.fcgi?cmd=Retrieve&db=pubmed&dopt=Abstract&list_uids=6226850

- **Osteopathy: improving the status of alternative healthcare.**
  Author(s): Drysdale I.
  Source: Occup Health (Lond). 1996 December; 48(12): 430-1. No Abstract Available.
  http://www.ncbi.nlm.nih.gov/entrez/query.fcgi?cmd=Retrieve&db=pubmed&dopt=Abstract&list_uids=9283456

- **Osteopathy: the 'orthodox' alternative.**
  Author(s): Stewart A.
  Source: Occup Health (Lond). 1992 May; 44(5): 152. No Abstract Available.
  http://www.ncbi.nlm.nih.gov/entrez/query.fcgi?cmd=Retrieve&db=pubmed&dopt=Abstract&list_uids=1285758

- **Osteopathy: the 'orthodox' alternative.**
  Author(s): Kaye J.
  Source: Occup Health (Lond). 1992 April; 44(4): 118-20.
  http://www.ncbi.nlm.nih.gov/entrez/query.fcgi?cmd=Retrieve&db=pubmed&dopt=Abstract&list_uids=1625846

- **Osteopathy--an aid to the healing process.**
  Author(s): Waldman P.
  Source: Prof Nurse. 1993 April; 8(7): 452-4.
  http://www.ncbi.nlm.nih.gov/entrez/query.fcgi?cmd=Retrieve&db=pubmed&dopt=Abstract&list_uids=8475150

- **Osteopathy--fifty years later. Founders Memorial Lecture. 1951.**
  Author(s): Fischer RL.
  Source: J Am Osteopath Assoc. 2001 January; 101(1): 43-8. No Abstract Available.
  http://www.ncbi.nlm.nih.gov/entrez/query.fcgi?cmd=Retrieve&db=pubmed&dopt=Abstract&list_uids=11236803

- **Patient confusion and misperception about the doctor of osteopathy and the medical doctor.**
  Author(s): Lindquist JD.
  Source: Journal of Health Care Marketing. 1988 March; 8(1): 76-81.
  http://www.ncbi.nlm.nih.gov/entrez/query.fcgi?cmd=Retrieve&db=pubmed&dopt=Abstract&list_uids=10286263

- **Post-radiation osteopathy.**
  Author(s): Salib PI.
  Source: Am J Orthop. 1964 May; 6(5): 122-5. No Abstract Available.
  http://www.ncbi.nlm.nih.gov/entrez/query.fcgi?cmd=Retrieve&db=pubmed&dopt=Abstract&list_uids=5875226

- **Radiological and histological improvement of oxalate osteopathy after combined liver-kidney transplantation in primary hyperoxaluria type 1.**
  Author(s): Toussaint C, De Pauw L, Vienne A, Gevenois PA, Quintin J, Gelin M, Pasteels JL.
  Source: American Journal of Kidney Diseases : the Official Journal of the National Kidney Foundation. 1993 January; 21(1): 54-63.
  http://www.ncbi.nlm.nih.gov/entrez/query.fcgi?cmd=Retrieve&db=pubmed&dopt=Abstract&list_uids=8418628

- **Rhabdomyolysis and severe haemolytic anaemia, hepatic dysfunction and intestinal osteopathy due to hypophosphataemia in a patient after Billroth II gastrectomy.**
  Author(s): Altuntas Y, Innice M, Basturk T, Seber S, Serin G, Ozturk B.
  Source: European Journal of Gastroenterology & Hepatology. 2002 May; 14(5): 555-7. Review.
  http://www.ncbi.nlm.nih.gov/entrez/query.fcgi?cmd=Retrieve&db=pubmed&dopt=Abstract&list_uids=11984155

- **Roentgen observations in diabetic osteopathy.**
  Author(s): Gondos B.
  Source: Radiology. 1968 July; 91(1): 6-13.
  http://www.ncbi.nlm.nih.gov/entrez/query.fcgi?cmd=Retrieve&db=pubmed&dopt=Abstract&list_uids=5654037

- **Role of keto acids in the prophylaxis and treatment of renal osteopathy.**
  Author(s): Frohling PT, Schmicker R, Lindenau K, Vetter K, Kokot F.
  Source: Contrib Nephrol. 1988; 65: 123-9.
  http://www.ncbi.nlm.nih.gov/entrez/query.fcgi?cmd=Retrieve&db=pubmed&dopt=Abstract&list_uids=3168459

- **Rose-colored view. The boom in osteopathy: what DOs are doing right.**
  Author(s): Peck P.
  Source: Physicians Manage. 1987 May; 27(5): 81-6, 89. No Abstract Available.
  http://www.ncbi.nlm.nih.gov/entrez/query.fcgi?cmd=Retrieve&db=pubmed&dopt=Abstract&list_uids=10282433

- **Saccharated ferric oxide-induced osteomalacia in Japan: iron-induced osteopathy due to nephropathy.**
  Author(s): Sato K, Shiraki M.
  Source: Endocrine Journal. 1998 August; 45(4): 431-9. Review.
  http://www.ncbi.nlm.nih.gov/entrez/query.fcgi?cmd=Retrieve&db=pubmed&dopt=Abstract&list_uids=9881891

- **Selected skeletal dysplasias: craniomandibular osteopathy, multiple cartilaginous exostoses, and hypertrophic osteodystrophy.**
  Author(s): Alexander JW.
  Source: The Veterinary Clinics of North America. Small Animal Practice. 1983 February; 13(1): 55-70. Review.
  http://www.ncbi.nlm.nih.gov/entrez/query.fcgi?cmd=Retrieve&db=pubmed&dopt=Abstract&list_uids=6346655

- **Severe arthropathy and osteopathy following combined renal/pancreas transplantation.**
  Author(s): Derfus BA, Carrera GF, Komorowski RA, Ryan LM.
  Source: Transplantation. 1992 March; 53(3): 678-81.
  http://www.ncbi.nlm.nih.gov/entrez/query.fcgi?cmd=Retrieve&db=pubmed&dopt=Abstract&list_uids=1549866

- **Spinal manipulation for low-back pain: a treatment package agreed to by the UK chiropractic, osteopathy and physiotherapy professional associations.**
  Author(s): Harvey E, Burton AK, Moffett JK, Breen A; UK BEAM trial team.
  Source: Manual Therapy. 2003 February; 8(1): 46-51. Review.
  http://www.ncbi.nlm.nih.gov/entrez/query.fcgi?cmd=Retrieve&db=pubmed&dopt=Abstract&list_uids=12635637

- **Sports injuries: how osteopathy can help.**
  Author(s): Moule TG.
  Source: Nursing (Lond). 1979 July; (4): 163-5. No Abstract Available.
  http://www.ncbi.nlm.nih.gov/entrez/query.fcgi?cmd=Retrieve&db=pubmed&dopt=Abstract&list_uids=161364

- **Stress osteopathy of the femoral head. 10 military recruits followed for 5-11 years.**
  Author(s): Visuri T.
  Source: Acta Orthopaedica Scandinavica. 1997 April; 68(2): 138-41.
  http://www.ncbi.nlm.nih.gov/entrez/query.fcgi?cmd=Retrieve&db=pubmed&dopt=Abstract&list_uids=9174450

- **Studies on psoriatic osteopathy.**
  Author(s): Hein G, Abendroth K, Muller A, Wessel G.
  Source: Clinical Rheumatology. 1991 March; 10(1): 13-7.
  http://www.ncbi.nlm.nih.gov/entrez/query.fcgi?cmd=Retrieve&db=pubmed&dopt=Abstract&list_uids=2065500

- **Study of the relationships between pericarditis and osteopathy in chronic haemodialysis.**
  Author(s): Mako J, Szucs J, Gaizler G, Lengyel M, Merei J.
  Source: International Urology and Nephrology. 1983; 15(4): 383-7.
  http://www.ncbi.nlm.nih.gov/entrez/query.fcgi?cmd=Retrieve&db=pubmed&dopt=Abstract&list_uids=6662655

- **The drive for professionalization in British osteopathy.**
  Author(s): Baer HA.
  Source: Social Science & Medicine (1982). 1984; 19(7): 717-25.
  http://www.ncbi.nlm.nih.gov/entrez/query.fcgi?cmd=Retrieve&db=pubmed&dopt=Abstract&list_uids=6548836

- **The organizational rejuvenation of osteopathy: a reflection of the decline of professional dominance in medicine.**
  Author(s): Baer HA.
  Source: Soc Sci Med [a]. 1981 September; 15(5): 701-11. No Abstract Available.
  http://www.ncbi.nlm.nih.gov/entrez/query.fcgi?cmd=Retrieve&db=pubmed&dopt=Abstract&list_uids=7034215

- **The paradox of osteopathy.**
  Author(s): Howell JD.
  Source: The New England Journal of Medicine. 1999 November 4; 341(19): 1465-8.
  http://www.ncbi.nlm.nih.gov/entrez/query.fcgi?cmd=Retrieve&db=pubmed&dopt=Abstract&list_uids=10547412

- **The treatment of uraemic osteopathy.**
  Author(s): Schaefer K, Schaefer P, Koeppe P, Opitz A, Hoffler D.
  Source: Ger Med Mon. 1969 May; 14(5): 238-40. No Abstract Available.
  http://www.ncbi.nlm.nih.gov/entrez/query.fcgi?cmd=Retrieve&db=pubmed&dopt=Abstract&list_uids=5820140

- **The treatment of uraemic osteopathy. II. The effect of 5,6-trans-25-hydroxycholecalciferol in terminal renal failure.**
  Author(s): von Herrath D, Kraft D, Grigoleit H, Schaefer K.
  Source: Ger Med. 1973 Winter; 3(3-4): 93-5. No Abstract Available.
  http://www.ncbi.nlm.nih.gov/entrez/query.fcgi?cmd=Retrieve&db=pubmed&dopt=Abstract&list_uids=4803059

- **Thomas L. Northup Lecture--1983 American Academy of Osteopathy: AAO--yesterday, today and tomorrow.**
  Author(s): Goodridge JP.
  Source: J Am Osteopath Assoc. 1984 April; 83(8): 593-600. No Abstract Available.
  http://www.ncbi.nlm.nih.gov/entrez/query.fcgi?cmd=Retrieve&db=pubmed&dopt=Abstract&list_uids=6547120

- **Thumbnail osteopathy.**
  Author(s): Handoll N.
  Source: J R Coll Gen Pract. 1984 July; 34(264): 409-11. No Abstract Available.
  http://www.ncbi.nlm.nih.gov/entrez/query.fcgi?cmd=Retrieve&db=pubmed&dopt=Abstract&list_uids=6547743

- **Unusual osteopathy in a newborn.**
  Author(s): Jequier S, Nogrady MB, Wesenberg RL.
  Source: Skeletal Radiology. 1983; 10(1): 20-5.
  http://www.ncbi.nlm.nih.gov/entrez/query.fcgi?cmd=Retrieve&db=pubmed&dopt=Abstract&list_uids=6879210

- **Uraemic osteopathy. The relationship between disturbances in intestinal calcium absorption and renal function.**
  Author(s): Schaefer K, Schaefer P, Koeppe P, Opitz A, Hoffler D.
  Source: Ger Med Mon. 1968 December; 13(12): 575-81. No Abstract Available.
  http://www.ncbi.nlm.nih.gov/entrez/query.fcgi?cmd=Retrieve&db=pubmed&dopt=Abstract&list_uids=5735338

- **Uremic osteopathy.**
  Author(s): Katic V, Dojcinov D, Strahinjic S, Savic V, Babic R, Markovic Z, Raicevic R.
  Source: Acta Med Iugosl. 1975; 29(3): 271-80. No Abstract Available.
  http://www.ncbi.nlm.nih.gov/entrez/query.fcgi?cmd=Retrieve&db=pubmed&dopt=Abstract&list_uids=1146605

- **Value of osteopathy.**
  Author(s): Miller JD.
  Source: British Medical Journal. 1970 September 26; 3(725): 772-3.
  http://www.ncbi.nlm.nih.gov/entrez/query.fcgi?cmd=Retrieve&db=pubmed&dopt=Abstract&list_uids=5536154

- **Widespread confusion prevails over 'osteopathy'.**
  Author(s): Truthan CE.
  Source: J Am Osteopath Assoc. 1998 December; 98(12): 674-5. No Abstract Available.
  http://www.ncbi.nlm.nih.gov/entrez/query.fcgi?cmd=Retrieve&db=pubmed&dopt=Abstract&list_uids=9885486

- **Women's health osteopathy: an alternative view.**
  Author(s): Hyne J.
  Source: Nursing Management (Harrow, London, England : 1994). 1998 December-1999 January; 5(8): 6-9.
  http://www.ncbi.nlm.nih.gov/entrez/query.fcgi?cmd=Retrieve&db=pubmed&dopt=Abstract&list_uids=10188493

- **X-ray photodensitometric analysis of anticonvulsant-induced osteopathy.**
  Author(s): Iwata Y, Amano K, Kawamura H, Tanikawa T, Kawabatake H, Notani M, Iseki H, Shiwaku T, Nagao T, Taira T, et al.
  Source: Jpn J Psychiatry Neurol. 1988 September; 42(3): 594-6. No Abstract Available.
  http://www.ncbi.nlm.nih.gov/entrez/query.fcgi?cmd=Retrieve&db=pubmed&dopt=Abstract&list_uids=3241486

CHAPTER 2. NUTRITION AND OSTEOPATHY

Overview

In this chapter, we will show you how to find studies dedicated specifically to nutrition and osteopathy.

Finding Nutrition Studies on Osteopathy

The National Institutes of Health's Office of Dietary Supplements (ODS) offers a searchable bibliographic database called the IBIDS (International Bibliographic Information on Dietary Supplements; National Institutes of Health, Building 31, Room 1B29, 31 Center Drive, MSC 2086, Bethesda, Maryland 20892-2086, Tel: 301-435-2920, Fax: 301-480-1845, E-mail: ods@nih.gov). The IBIDS contains over 460,000 scientific citations and summaries about dietary supplements and nutrition as well as references to published international, scientific literature on dietary supplements such as vitamins, minerals, and botanicals.[7] The IBIDS includes references and citations to both human and animal research studies.

As a service of the ODS, access to the IBIDS database is available free of charge at the following Web address: **http://ods.od.nih.gov/databases/ibids.html**. After entering the search area, you have three choices: (1) IBIDS Consumer Database, (2) Full IBIDS Database, or (3) Peer Reviewed Citations Only.

Now that you have selected a database, click on the "Advanced" tab. An advanced search allows you to retrieve up to 100 fully explained references in a comprehensive format. Type "osteopathy" (or synonyms) into the search box, and click "Go." To narrow the search, you can also select the "Title" field.

---

[7] Adapted from **http://ods.od.nih.gov**. IBIDS is produced by the Office of Dietary Supplements (ODS) at the National Institutes of Health to assist the public, healthcare providers, educators, and researchers in locating credible, scientific information on dietary supplements. IBIDS was developed and will be maintained through an interagency partnership with the Food and Nutrition Information Center of the National Agricultural Library, U.S. Department of Agriculture.

The following information is typical of that found when using the "Full IBIDS Database" to search for "osteopathy" (or a synonym):

- **Hypertrophic osteopathy and pneumonia in a macropod.**
  Author(s): Department of Veterinary Pathology and Anatomy, School of Veterinary Science and Animal Production, University of Queensland.
  Source: Wayne, J Nicholson, V Aust-Vet-J. 1999 February; 77(2): 98-9 0005-0423

Federal Resources on Nutrition

In addition to the IBIDS, the United States Department of Health and Human Services (HHS) and the United States Department of Agriculture (USDA) provide many sources of information on general nutrition and health. Recommended resources include:

- healthfinder®, HHS's gateway to health information, including diet and nutrition: **http://www.healthfinder.gov/scripts/SearchContext.asp?topic=238&page=0**

- The United States Department of Agriculture's Web site dedicated to nutrition information: **www.nutrition.gov**

- The Food and Drug Administration's Web site for federal food safety information: **www.foodsafety.gov**

- The National Action Plan on Overweight and Obesity sponsored by the United States Surgeon General: **http://www.surgeongeneral.gov/topics/obesity/**

- The Center for Food Safety and Applied Nutrition has an Internet site sponsored by the Food and Drug Administration and the Department of Health and Human Services: **http://vm.cfsan.fda.gov/**

- Center for Nutrition Policy and Promotion sponsored by the United States Department of Agriculture: **http://www.usda.gov/cnpp/**

- Food and Nutrition Information Center, National Agricultural Library sponsored by the United States Department of Agriculture: **http://www.nal.usda.gov/fnic/**

- Food and Nutrition Service sponsored by the United States Department of Agriculture: **http://www.fns.usda.gov/fns/**

Additional Web Resources

A number of additional Web sites offer encyclopedic information covering food and nutrition. The following is a representative sample:

- AOL: **http://search.aol.com/cat.adp?id=174&layer=&from=subcats**

- Family Village: **http://www.familyvillage.wisc.edu/med_nutrition.html**

- Google: **http://directory.google.com/Top/Health/Nutrition/**

- Healthnotes: **http://www.healthnotes.com/**

- Open Directory Project: **http://dmoz.org/Health/Nutrition/**

- Yahoo.com: **http://dir.yahoo.com/Health/Nutrition/**

- WebMD®Health: **http://my.webmd.com/nutrition**

- WholeHealthMD.com: **http://www.wholehealthmd.com/reflib/0,1529,00.html**

CHAPTER 3. ALTERNATIVE MEDICINE AND OSTEOPATHY

Overview

In this chapter, we will begin by introducing you to official information sources on complementary and alternative medicine (CAM) relating to osteopathy. At the conclusion of this chapter, we will provide additional sources.

The Combined Health Information Database

The Combined Health Information Database (CHID) is a bibliographic database produced by health-related agencies of the U.S. federal government (mostly from the National Institutes of Health) that can offer concise information for a targeted search. The CHID database is updated four times a year at the end of January, April, July, and October. Check the titles, summaries, and availability of CAM-related information by using the "Simple Search" option at the following Web site: **http://chid.nih.gov/simple/simple.html**. In the drop box at the top, select "Complementary and Alternative Medicine." Then type "osteopathy" (or synonyms) in the second search box. We recommend that you select 100 "documents per page" and to check the "whole records" options. The following was extracted using this technique:

- **Alternative Medicine Online: A Guide to Natural Remedies on the Internet**

  Source: Blue Ridge Summit, PA: National Book Network. 1997. 216 p.

  Contact: Available from National Book Network. P.O. Box 190, Blue Ridge Summit, PA 17214. (800) 462-6420. PRICE: $12.95. ISBN: 1881025101.

  Summary: This book is a guide to alternative medicine on the Internet. The author describes more than 50 world-wide web sites that contain information about alternative medicine. The book details useful and sometimes offbeat sites on-line. Chapters are organized alphabetically by topics including acupuncture, apitherapy, Eye Movement Desensitizing and Reprocessing (EMDR), gemstones, Richard Evans, M.D.; **osteopathy, Ontario guide; Sunsite; Wound Care Institute;** and Andrew Weil. Each section contains the web site title, address, information, and the author's opinion about whether or not it is helpful. The book contains an index to topics and graphics of the actual web site.

- **AMA Report of the Council on Scientific Affairs on Alternative Medicine**

  Source: Townsend Letter for Doctors and Patients. Number 178: 135-145. January 1998.

  Summary: This journal article reports on the American Medical Association (AMA) Report of the Council on Scientific Affairs on Alternative Medicine. Several alternative systems and techniques are defined, including mind/body interventions, diet and nutrition, herbal remedies, **osteopathy,** chiropractic, energy healing, pharmacologic methods, acupuncture, homeopathy, naturopathy, Ayurveda, and folk therapies. The Office of Alternative Medicine and the context of the public's use of alternative medicine are discussed. The Council on Scientific Affairs makes several recommendations for dealing with alternative medicine, including (1) promoting well-designed, stringently controlled research studies to determine the efficacy of alternative therapies, (2) urging physicians to inquire routinely about their patients' use of alternative medicine and to educate themselves and their patients on the state of scientific knowledge on alternative therapy, and (3) urging medical schools to offer courses on alternative medicine that will present scientific views of unconventional theories, treatments, and practice as well as the potential therapeutic utility, safety, and efficacy of these modalities. Finally, the Council recommends that patients choosing alternative therapies should be educated as to the hazards that might result from postponing or stopping conventional medical treatments. This journal article contains 39 references.

National Center for Complementary and Alternative Medicine

The National Center for Complementary and Alternative Medicine (NCCAM) of the National Institutes of Health (**http://nccam.nih.gov/**) has created a link to the National Library of Medicine's databases to facilitate research for articles that specifically relate to osteopathy and complementary medicine. To search the database, go to the following Web site: **http://www.nlm.nih.gov/nccam/camonpubmed.html**. Select "CAM on PubMed." Enter "osteopathy" (or synonyms) into the search box. Click "Go." The following references provide information on particular aspects of complementary and alternative medicine that are related to osteopathy:

- **"Failed conservative care": always define what treatment was received.**
  Author(s): Mooney V.
  Source: The Spine Journal : Official Journal of the North American Spine Society. 2001 March-April; 1(2): 159; Discussion 160.
  http://www.ncbi.nlm.nih.gov/entrez/query.fcgi?cmd=Retrieve&db=pubmed&dopt=Abstract&list_uids=14588405

- **Cardiogenic hypertrophic osteopathy in a dog with a right-to-left shunting patent ductus arteriosus.**
  Author(s): Anderson TP, Walker MC, Goring RL.
  Source: J Am Vet Med Assoc. 2004 May 1; 224(9): 1464-6, 1453.
  http://www.ncbi.nlm.nih.gov/entrez/query.fcgi?cmd=Retrieve&db=pubmed&dopt=Abstract&list_uids=15124887

- **Study raises important issues about the potential benefit of osteopathy in the cranial field to patients with Parkinson's disease.**
  Author(s): Boehm KM, Lawner BJ, McFee RB.

Source: J Am Osteopath Assoc. 2003 August; 103(8): 354-5; Author Reply 355-6. No Abstract Available.
http://www.ncbi.nlm.nih.gov/entrez/query.fcgi?cmd=Retrieve&db=pubmed&dopt=Abstract&list_uids=12956246

Additional Web Resources

A number of additional Web sites offer encyclopedic information covering CAM and related topics. The following is a representative sample:

- Alternative Medicine Foundation, Inc.: **http://www.herbmed.org/**

- AOL: **http://search.aol.com/cat.adp?id=169&layer=&from=subcats**

- Chinese Medicine: **http://www.newcenturynutrition.com/**

- drkoop.com®: **http://www.drkoop.com/InteractiveMedicine/IndexC.html**

- Family Village: **http://www.familyvillage.wisc.edu/med_altn.htm**

- Google: **http://directory.google.com/Top/Health/Alternative/**

- Healthnotes: **http://www.healthnotes.com/**

- MedWebPlus:
  http://medwebplus.com/subject/Alternative_and_Complementary_Medicine

- Open Directory Project: **http://dmoz.org/Health/Alternative/**

- HealthGate: **http://www.tnp.com/**

- WebMD®Health: **http://my.webmd.com/drugs_and_herbs**

- WholeHealthMD.com: **http://www.wholehealthmd.com/reflib/0,1529,00.html**

- Yahoo.com: **http://dir.yahoo.com/Health/Alternative_Medicine/**

The following is a specific Web list relating to osteopathy; please note that any particular subject below may indicate either a therapeutic use, or a contraindication (potential danger), and does not reflect an official recommendation:

- **General Overview**

  Migraine Headaches
  Source: Healthnotes, Inc.; www.healthnotes.com

- **Alternative Therapy**

  Acupuncture
  Source: WholeHealthMD.com, LLC.; www.wholehealthmd.com
  Hyperlink:
  http://www.wholehealthmd.com/refshelf/substances_view/0,1525,663,00.html

Acupuncture Osteopathy
Source: The Canoe version of A Dictionary of Alternative-Medicine Methods, by Priorities for Health editor Jack Raso, M.S., R.D.
Hyperlink: http://www.canoe.ca/AltmedDictionary/a.html

Bodywork
Alternative names: Bodywork Therapy
Source: The Canoe version of A Dictionary of Alternative-Medicine Methods, by Priorities for Health editor Jack Raso, M.S., R.D.
Hyperlink: http://www.canoe.ca/AltmedDictionary/b.html

Chelation Therapy
Source: WholeHealthMD.com, LLC.; www.wholehealthmd.com
Hyperlink:
http://www.wholehealthmd.com/refshelf/substances_view/0,1525,679,00.html

Chiropractic
Source: WholeHealthMD.com, LLC.; www.wholehealthmd.com
Hyperlink:
http://www.wholehealthmd.com/refshelf/substances_view/0,1525,681,00.html

Craniosacral Therapy
Alternative names: cranial balancing cranial osteopathy cranial sacral manipulation cranial technique cranial work craniopathy craniosacral balancing Craniosacral Osteopathy Cranio-Sacral work
Source: The Canoe version of A Dictionary of Alternative-Medicine Methods, by Priorities for Health editor Jack Raso, M.S., R.D.
Hyperlink: http://www.canoe.ca/AltmedDictionary/c.html

Craniosacral Therapy
Source: WholeHealthMD.com, LLC.; www.wholehealthmd.com
Hyperlink:
http://www.wholehealthmd.com/refshelf/substances_view/0,1525,685,00.html

Fasting
Source: WholeHealthMD.com, LLC.; www.wholehealthmd.com
Hyperlink:
http://www.wholehealthmd.com/refshelf/substances_view/0,1525,694,00.html

Neural Organization Technique
Alternative names: NOT
Source: The Canoe version of A Dictionary of Alternative-Medicine Methods, by Priorities for Health editor Jack Raso, M.S., R.D.
Hyperlink: http://www.canoe.ca/AltmedDictionary/n.html

Osteopathy
Source: Integrative Medicine Communications; www.drkoop.com

Osteopathy
Source: WholeHealthMD.com, LLC.; www.wholehealthmd.com
Hyperlink:
http://www.wholehealthmd.com/refshelf/substances_view/0,1525,724,00.html

Polarity Therapy
Source: WholeHealthMD.com, LLC.; www.wholehealthmd.com
Hyperlink:
http://www.wholehealthmd.com/refshelf/substances_view/0,1525,727,00.html

Rolfing
Source: WholeHealthMD.com, LLC.; www.wholehealthmd.com
Hyperlink:
http://www.wholehealthmd.com/refshelf/substances_view/0,1525,732,00.html

General References

A good place to find general background information on CAM is the National Library of Medicine. It has prepared within the MEDLINEplus system an information topic page dedicated to complementary and alternative medicine. To access this page, go to the MEDLINEplus site at **http://www.nlm.nih.gov/medlineplus/alternativemedicine.html**. This Web site provides a general overview of various topics and can lead to a number of general sources.

CHAPTER 4. PATENTS ON OSTEOPATHY

Overview

Patents can be physical innovations (e.g. chemicals, pharmaceuticals, medical equipment) or processes (e.g. treatments or diagnostic procedures). The United States Patent and Trademark Office defines a patent as a grant of a property right to the inventor, issued by the Patent and Trademark Office.[8] Patents, therefore, are intellectual property. For the United States, the term of a new patent is 20 years from the date when the patent application was filed. If the inventor wishes to receive economic benefits, it is likely that the invention will become commercially available within 20 years of the initial filing. It is important to understand, therefore, that an inventor's patent does not indicate that a product or service is or will be commercially available. The patent implies only that the inventor has "the right to exclude others from making, using, offering for sale, or selling" the invention in the United States. While this relates to U.S. patents, similar rules govern foreign patents.

In this chapter, we show you how to locate information on patents and their inventors. If you find a patent that is particularly interesting to you, contact the inventor or the assignee for further information. **IMPORTANT NOTE:** When following the search strategy described below, you may discover non-medical patents that use the generic term "osteopathy" (or a synonym) in their titles. To accurately reflect the results that you might find while conducting research on osteopathy, we have not necessarily excluded non-medical patents in this bibliography.

Patents on Osteopathy

By performing a patent search focusing on osteopathy, you can obtain information such as the title of the invention, the names of the inventor(s), the assignee(s) or the company that owns or controls the patent, a short abstract that summarizes the patent, and a few excerpts from the description of the patent. The abstract of a patent tends to be more technical in nature, while the description is often written for the public. Full patent descriptions contain much more information than is presented here (e.g. claims, references, figures, diagrams, etc.). We will tell you how to obtain this information later in the chapter. The following is an

---

[8]Adapted from the United States Patent and Trademark Office:
http://www.uspto.gov/web/offices/pac/doc/general/whatis.htm.

example of the type of information that you can expect to obtain from a patent search on osteopathy:

- **Peptides and remedy for bone diseases containing the same as active ingredient**

    Inventor(s): Sakamoto; Kenji (25, Aza Kourokuzawa, Memeki, Yuuwa-machi, Kawabe-gun, Akita 010-12, JP)

    Assignee(s): none reported

    Patent Number: 6,071,881

    Date filed: January 4, 1999

    Abstract: A new substance useful as a drug for the treatment of **osteopathy** is disclosed. The present invention provides a peptide and derivative thereof, the peptide having an amino acid sequence SEQ ID NO:1 designated hereunder as follows, wherein both of the peptide and derivative thereof having growth promotion effects and activity promotion effects on osteoblasts, as well as a drug having the peptide as an effective component for the treatment of osteopathy:

    Excerpt(s): The present invention relates to a new drug containing the same as an effective component for treating **osteopathy.** It is well known that there are a number of physiological active substances in a human body, and that such substances are closely involved in the support of normal biological activities in a human body. Both of such physiological active substances of a human body and synthesized physiological active substances are showing possibilities of being new drugs as well as providing new insights into the development of new drugs. Therefore, the search for such physiological active substances is of utmost importance. On the other hand, for the treatment of **osteopathy** such as osteoporosis, calcitonin, female hormone, and activated vitamin D3 and the like are currently used, the remedial effects thereof are not necessarily of satisfactory one.

    Web site: http://www.delphion.com/details?pn=US06071881__

Patent Applications on Osteopathy

As of December 2000, U.S. patent applications are open to public viewing.[9] Applications are patent requests which have yet to be granted. (The process to achieve a patent can take several years.) The following patent applications have been filed since December 2000 relating to osteopathy:

- **Dynamic computing imagery, especially for visceral osteopathy and for articular kinetics**

    Inventor(s): Finet, Georges; (Quaregnon, BE), Williame, Christian; (Quaregnon, BE)

    Correspondence: Hovey Williams Timmons & Collins; 2405 Grand BLVD., Suite 400; Kansas City; MO; 64108

    Patent Application Number: 20030081837

    Date filed: June 10, 2002

---

[9] This has been a common practice outside the United States prior to December 2000.

Abstract: Computerized method for studying alterations in the location of an object, said method comprising the steps of computing successive shapes by means of a dynamic contour model algorithm, whereby the dynamic contour model algorithm develops successive shapes and determines a correlation between two successive shapes and for stopping the reiteration of the algorithm when said determined correlation is lower than a predetermined value.

Excerpt(s): This application is a continuation-in-part of co-pending International Application No. PCT/BE00/00145, with an international filing date of Dec. 8, 2000, published in English under PCT Article 21(2) on Jun. 14, 2001 which claims the benefit of U.S. Provisional Application No. 60/170,222 filed Dec. 10, 1999. The present invention is related to a computing imagery method for studying alterations in the location of an object after a movement thereof. In said method, the position of the object in two images is analyzed. This method is particularly suitable for evaluating or controlling visceral movement or articular kinetics based on medical imaging techniques. The invention is equally related to a computer program for performing said method. It has already been proposed to analyze two images of an object so as to determine the movement of said object between its position in the first image and its position in its second image.

Web site: http://appft1.uspto.gov/netahtml/PTO/search-bool.html

- **Novel peptides and remedy for bone diseases containing the same as active ingredient**

Inventor(s): Sakamoto, Kenji; (Kawabe-gun, JP)

Correspondence: James N. Kallis; Brooks & Kushman P.C.; 22nd Floor; 1000 Town Center; Southfield; MI; 48075-1351; US

Patent Application Number: 20040162415

Date filed: March 11, 2002

Abstract: A new substance useful as a drug for the treatment of **osteopathy** is disclosed. The present invention provides a peptide and derivative thereof, said peptide having an amino acid sequence SEQ ID NO: 1 designated hereunder as follows, wherein both of the peptide and derivative thereof having growth promotion effects and activity promotion effects on osteoblasts, as well as a drug having the peptide as an effective component for the treatment of osteopathy: 1 SEQ ID NO: 1 Lys Leu Thr Thr Ile Phe Pro Leu Asn Trp 1 5 10 Lys Tyr Arg Lys Ala Leu. 15

Excerpt(s): This is a continuation of copending application Ser. No. 08/930,776, filed on Jan. 4, 1999, entitled, "Novel Peptides and Remedy for Bone Diseases Containing the Same as Active Ingredient". The present invention relates to a new drug containing the same as an effective component for treating **osteopathy**. It is well known that there are a number of physiological active substances in a human body, and that such substances are closely involved in the support of normal biological activities in a human body. Both of such physiological active substances of a human body and synthesized physiological active substances are showing possibilities of being new drugs as well as providing new insights into the development of new drugs. Therefore, the search for such physiological active substances is of utmost importance.

Web site: http://appft1.uspto.gov/netahtml/PTO/search-bool.html

- **PROCESS OF MAKING AN OSTEOPATHY SOLUTION**

Inventor(s): Zuo, Xiao-Feng; (Shanghai, CN)

Correspondence: Raymond Y. Chan; 108 N.YNEZ AVE. Suite 128; Monterey Park; CA; 91754; US

Patent Application Number: 20040013750

Date filed: July 16, 2002

Abstract: A process of making an **osteopathy** solution includes the steps of (a) soaking a raw composition which includes Radix Angelicae Sinensis, Radix Paeoniae Rubra, Rhizoma seu Radix Notopterygii, Radix Angelicae Dahuricae, Herba Asari, Folium Artemisiae Argyi, Radix Angelicae Pubescentis, Radix Dipsaci, Myrrha, Ramulus Mori, Radix Rubiae, Radix Clematidis, Radix Stephaniae Tetrandrae, Rhizoma Cimicifugae and Radix Gentianae Macrophyllae in a predetermined amount of water for a predetermined period of soaking time to form a pre-decocting solution and a pre-decocting composition; (b) heating the pre-decocting solution and the pre-decocting composition for a predetermined period of reaction time to form a mixture consisting of a residual composition and a solution; wherein a volume ratio of said solution in step (b) and said water in step (a) is approximately 1:3; and (c) cooling down the solution to a predetermined temperature.

Excerpt(s): The present invention relates to a process of making an **osteopathy** solution, and more particularly to an **osteopathy** solution for promoting the process of natural healing activities of human bodies. Health is a kind of balance of our bodies and the environment. Any forms of imbalance in our bodies will initiate the generation of signals from our bodies. Proper reaction should be done for the signal to restore our bodies to normal. If we neglect the signals from our bodies, we will gradually feel uncomfortable and eventually get sick. The importance of balance of our bodies can be easily shown in our daily lives. For example, when our bodies suffer from deficiency of water, we will feel thirsty. The sense of feeling thirsty is a signal from our bodies to alert us the necessity of drinking water for restoring the balance of our bodies. Therefore, when we receive the signal of feeling thirsty, we may act by drinking water to restore the osmosis of our bodies to normal. However, if we ignore the signal, the level of deficiency of water will gradually increase and our bodies will become very uncomfortable. Under prolonged situation of suffering water deficiency, we will start to get sick and will eventually die of dehydration.

Web site: http://appft1.uspto.gov/netahtml/PTO/search-bool.html

Keeping Current

In order to stay informed about patents and patent applications dealing with osteopathy, you can access the U.S. Patent Office archive via the Internet at the following Web address: **http://www.uspto.gov/patft/index.html**. You will see two broad options: (1) Issued Patent, and (2) Published Applications. To see a list of issued patents, perform the following steps: Under "Issued Patents," click "Quick Search." Then, type "osteopathy" (or synonyms) into the "Term 1" box. After clicking on the search button, scroll down to see the various patents which have been granted to date on osteopathy.

You can also use this procedure to view pending patent applications concerning osteopathy. Simply go back to **http://www.uspto.gov/patft/index.html**. Select "Quick Search" under "Published Applications." Then proceed with the steps listed above.

CHAPTER 5. BOOKS ON OSTEOPATHY

Overview

This chapter provides bibliographic book references relating to osteopathy. In addition to online booksellers such as **www.amazon.com** and **www.bn.com**, excellent sources for book titles on osteopathy include the Combined Health Information Database and the National Library of Medicine. Your local medical library also may have these titles available for loan.

Book Summaries: Federal Agencies

The Combined Health Information Database collects various book abstracts from a variety of healthcare institutions and federal agencies. To access these summaries, go directly to the following hyperlink: **http://chid.nih.gov/detail/detail.html**. You will need to use the "Detailed Search" option. To find book summaries, use the drop boxes at the bottom of the search page where "You may refine your search by." Select the dates and language you prefer. For the format option, select "Monograph/Book." Now type "osteopathy" (or synonyms) into the "For these words:" box. You should check back periodically with this database which is updated every three months. The following is a typical result when searching for books on osteopathy:

- **Staying Healthy With HIV: A Guide to Alternative and Complementary Therapies**

  Contact: Richard Copeland, 273 A State St, San Francisco, CA, 94114, (415) 255-2327.

  Summary: This book presents a guide to therapeutic treatments for HIV-positive people. It discusses stress management methods; nutrition and nutrition supplements; understanding blood test results; alternative therapies, such as acupuncture and **osteopathy;** FDA-approved treatments; experimental treatments, including immune modulators; choosing a treatment plan; and a recommended standard of care. The book also contains a resource guide and worksheets.

Book Summaries: Online Booksellers

Commercial Internet-based booksellers, such as Amazon.com and Barnes&Noble.com, offer summaries which have been supplied by each title's publisher. Some summaries also include customer reviews. Your local bookseller may have access to in-house and commercial databases that index all published books (e.g. Books in Print®). **IMPORTANT NOTE:** Online booksellers typically produce search results for medical and non-medical books. When searching for "osteopathy" at online booksellers' Web sites, you may discover non-medical books that use the generic term "osteopathy" (or a synonym) in their titles. The following is indicative of the results you might find when searching for "osteopathy" (sorted alphabetically by title; follow the hyperlink to view more details at Amazon.com):

- **A guide to osteopathy (New ways to health)** by Stephen Sandler; ISBN: 0600560139; http://www.amazon.com/exec/obidos/ASIN/0600560139/icongroupinterna

- **A New American Acupuncture : Acupuncture Osteopathy : The Myofascial Release of the Bodymind's** by Mark Seem; ISBN: 0936185449; http://www.amazon.com/exec/obidos/ASIN/0936185449/icongroupinterna

- **Autobiography of Andrew T. Still, With a History of the Discovery and Development of the Science of Osteopathy (Medicine & Society in America)** by A. T. Still; ISBN: 0405039735; http://www.amazon.com/exec/obidos/ASIN/0405039735/icongroupinterna

- **Early Osteopathy in the Words of A.T. Still, Illustrated** by Andrew Taylor Still, R.V. Schnucker; ISBN: 0943549116; http://www.amazon.com/exec/obidos/ASIN/0943549116/icongroupinterna

- **Healing with Osteopathy (Healing with)** by Peta Sneddon, Paolo Cosechi; ISBN: 0717124649; http://www.amazon.com/exec/obidos/ASIN/0717124649/icongroupinterna

- **History of Osteopathy and Twenty Century Medical Practice** by Emmons Rutledge Booth; ISBN: 0404134017; http://www.amazon.com/exec/obidos/ASIN/0404134017/icongroupinterna

- **Orthopathic Medicine: The Unification of Orthopedics With Osteopathy Through the Facial Distortion Model** by Stephen Typaldos; ISBN: 0965964124; http://www.amazon.com/exec/obidos/ASIN/0965964124/icongroupinterna

- **The central connection: Somatovisceral/viscerosomatic interaction : proceedings of the 1989 American Academy of Osteopathy International Symposium** by American Academy of Osteopathy; ISBN: 0914127292; http://www.amazon.com/exec/obidos/ASIN/0914127292/icongroupinterna

- **The collected papers of Viola M. Frymann : legacy of osteopathy to children** by Viola M. Frymann; ISBN: 0940668084; http://www.amazon.com/exec/obidos/ASIN/0940668084/icongroupinterna

APPENDICES

APPENDIX A. PHYSICIAN RESOURCES

Overview

In this chapter, we focus on databases and Internet-based guidelines and information resources created or written for a professional audience.

NIH Guidelines

Commonly referred to as "clinical" or "professional" guidelines, the National Institutes of Health publish physician guidelines for the most common diseases. Publications are available at the following by relevant Institute[10]:

- Office of the Director (OD); guidelines consolidated across agencies available at **http://www.nih.gov/health/consumer/conkey.htm**

- National Institute of General Medical Sciences (NIGMS); fact sheets available at **http://www.nigms.nih.gov/news/facts/**

- National Library of Medicine (NLM); extensive encyclopedia (A.D.A.M., Inc.) with guidelines: **http://www.nlm.nih.gov/medlineplus/healthtopics.html**

- National Cancer Institute (NCI); guidelines available at **http://www.cancer.gov/cancerinfo/list.aspx?viewid=5f35036e-5497-4d86-8c2c-714a9f7c8d25**

- National Eye Institute (NEI); guidelines available at **http://www.nei.nih.gov/order/index.htm**

- National Heart, Lung, and Blood Institute (NHLBI); guidelines available at **http://www.nhlbi.nih.gov/guidelines/index.htm**

- National Human Genome Research Institute (NHGRI); research available at **http://www.genome.gov/page.cfm?pageID=10000375**

- National Institute on Aging (NIA); guidelines available at **http://www.nia.nih.gov/health/**

---

[10] These publications are typically written by one or more of the various NIH Institutes.

- National Institute on Alcohol Abuse and Alcoholism (NIAAA); guidelines available at http://www.niaaa.nih.gov/publications/publications.htm

- National Institute of Allergy and Infectious Diseases (NIAID); guidelines available at http://www.niaid.nih.gov/publications/

- National Institute of Arthritis and Musculoskeletal and Skin Diseases (NIAMS); fact sheets and guidelines available at http://www.niams.nih.gov/hi/index.htm

- National Institute of Child Health and Human Development (NICHD); guidelines available at http://www.nichd.nih.gov/publications/pubskey.cfm

- National Institute on Deafness and Other Communication Disorders (NIDCD); fact sheets and guidelines at http://www.nidcd.nih.gov/health/

- National Institute of Dental and Craniofacial Research (NIDCR); guidelines available at http://www.nidr.nih.gov/health/

- National Institute of Diabetes and Digestive and Kidney Diseases (NIDDK); guidelines available at http://www.niddk.nih.gov/health/health.htm

- National Institute on Drug Abuse (NIDA); guidelines available at http://www.nida.nih.gov/DrugAbuse.html

- National Institute of Environmental Health Sciences (NIEHS); environmental health information available at http://www.niehs.nih.gov/external/facts.htm

- National Institute of Mental Health (NIMH); guidelines available at http://www.nimh.nih.gov/practitioners/index.cfm

- National Institute of Neurological Disorders and Stroke (NINDS); neurological disorder information pages available at http://www.ninds.nih.gov/health_and_medical/disorder_index.htm

- National Institute of Nursing Research (NINR); publications on selected illnesses at http://www.nih.gov/ninr/news-info/publications.html

- National Institute of Biomedical Imaging and Bioengineering; general information at http://grants.nih.gov/grants/becon/becon_info.htm

- Center for Information Technology (CIT); referrals to other agencies based on keyword searches available at http://kb.nih.gov/www_query_main.asp

- National Center for Complementary and Alternative Medicine (NCCAM); health information available at http://nccam.nih.gov/health/

- National Center for Research Resources (NCRR); various information directories available at http://www.ncrr.nih.gov/publications.asp

- Office of Rare Diseases; various fact sheets available at http://rarediseases.info.nih.gov/html/resources/rep_pubs.html

- Centers for Disease Control and Prevention; various fact sheets on infectious diseases available at http://www.cdc.gov/publications.htm

NIH Databases

In addition to the various Institutes of Health that publish professional guidelines, the NIH has designed a number of databases for professionals.[11] Physician-oriented resources provide a wide variety of information related to the biomedical and health sciences, both past and present. The format of these resources varies. Searchable databases, bibliographic citations, full-text articles (when available), archival collections, and images are all available. The following are referenced by the National Library of Medicine:[12]

- **Bioethics:** Access to published literature on the ethical, legal, and public policy issues surrounding healthcare and biomedical research. This information is provided in conjunction with the Kennedy Institute of Ethics located at Georgetown University, Washington, D.C.: **http://www.nlm.nih.gov/databases/databases_bioethics.html**

- **HIV/AIDS Resources:** Describes various links and databases dedicated to HIV/AIDS research: **http://www.nlm.nih.gov/pubs/factsheets/aidsinfs.html**

- **NLM Online Exhibitions:** Describes "Exhibitions in the History of Medicine": **http://www.nlm.nih.gov/exhibition/exhibition.html**. Additional resources for historical scholarship in medicine: **http://www.nlm.nih.gov/hmd/hmd.html**

- **Biotechnology Information:** Access to public databases. The National Center for Biotechnology Information conducts research in computational biology, develops software tools for analyzing genome data, and disseminates biomedical information for the better understanding of molecular processes affecting human health and disease: **http://www.ncbi.nlm.nih.gov/**

- **Population Information:** The National Library of Medicine provides access to worldwide coverage of population, family planning, and related health issues, including family planning technology and programs, fertility, and population law and policy: **http://www.nlm.nih.gov/databases/databases_population.html**

- **Cancer Information:** Access to cancer-oriented databases: **http://www.nlm.nih.gov/databases/databases_cancer.html**

- **Profiles in Science:** Offering the archival collections of prominent twentieth-century biomedical scientists to the public through modern digital technology: **http://www.profiles.nlm.nih.gov/**

- **Chemical Information:** Provides links to various chemical databases and references: **http://sis.nlm.nih.gov/Chem/ChemMain.html**

- **Clinical Alerts:** Reports the release of findings from the NIH-funded clinical trials where such release could significantly affect morbidity and mortality: **http://www.nlm.nih.gov/databases/alerts/clinical_alerts.html**

- **Space Life Sciences:** Provides links and information to space-based research (including NASA): **http://www.nlm.nih.gov/databases/databases_space.html**

- **MEDLINE:** Bibliographic database covering the fields of medicine, nursing, dentistry, veterinary medicine, the healthcare system, and the pre-clinical sciences: **http://www.nlm.nih.gov/databases/databases_medline.html**

---

[11] Remember, for the general public, the National Library of Medicine recommends the databases referenced in MEDLINE*plus* (**http://medlineplus.gov/** or **http://www.nlm.nih.gov/medlineplus/databases.html**).

[12] See **http://www.nlm.nih.gov/databases/databases.html**.

- **Toxicology and Environmental Health Information (TOXNET):** Databases covering toxicology and environmental health: **http://sis.nlm.nih.gov/Tox/ToxMain.html**

- **Visible Human Interface:** Anatomically detailed, three-dimensional representations of normal male and female human bodies:
  http://www.nlm.nih.gov/research/visible/visible_human.html

The NLM Gateway[13]

The NLM (National Library of Medicine) Gateway is a Web-based system that lets users search simultaneously in multiple retrieval systems at the U.S. National Library of Medicine (NLM). It allows users of NLM services to initiate searches from one Web interface, providing one-stop searching for many of NLM's information resources or databases.[14] To use the NLM Gateway, simply go to the search site at **http://gateway.nlm.nih.gov/gw/Cmd**. Type "osteopathy" (or synonyms) into the search box and click "Search." The results will be presented in a tabular form, indicating the number of references in each database category.

Results Summary

Category	Items Found
Journal Articles	247714
Books / Periodicals / Audio Visual	4900
Consumer Health	762
Meeting Abstracts	11
Other Collections	6
Total	253393

HSTAT[15]

HSTAT is a free, Web-based resource that provides access to full-text documents used in healthcare decision-making.[16] These documents include clinical practice guidelines, quick-reference guides for clinicians, consumer health brochures, evidence reports and technology assessments from the Agency for Healthcare Research and Quality (AHRQ), as well as AHRQ's Put Prevention Into Practice.[17] Simply search by "osteopathy" (or synonyms) at the following Web site: **http://text.nlm.nih.gov**.

---

[13] Adapted from NLM: **http://gateway.nlm.nih.gov/gw/Cmd?Overview.x**.

[14] The NLM Gateway is currently being developed by the Lister Hill National Center for Biomedical Communications (LHNCBC) at the National Library of Medicine (NLM) of the National Institutes of Health (NIH).

[15] Adapted from HSTAT: **http://www.nlm.nih.gov/pubs/factsheets/hstat.html**.

[16] The HSTAT URL is **http://hstat.nlm.nih.gov/**.

[17] Other important documents in HSTAT include: the National Institutes of Health (NIH) Consensus Conference Reports and Technology Assessment Reports; the HIV/AIDS Treatment Information Service (ATIS) resource documents; the Substance Abuse and Mental Health Services Administration's Center for Substance Abuse Treatment (SAMHSA/CSAT) Treatment Improvement Protocols (TIP) and Center for Substance Abuse Prevention (SAMHSA/CSAP) Prevention Enhancement Protocols System (PEPS); the Public Health Service (PHS) Preventive Services Task Force's *Guide to Clinical Preventive Services*; the independent, nonfederal Task Force on Community Services' *Guide to Community Preventive Services*; and the Health Technology Advisory Committee (HTAC) of the Minnesota Health Care Commission (MHCC) health technology evaluations.

Coffee Break: Tutorials for Biologists[18]

Coffee Break is a general healthcare site that takes a scientific view of the news and covers recent breakthroughs in biology that may one day assist physicians in developing treatments. Here you will find a collection of short reports on recent biological discoveries. Each report incorporates interactive tutorials that demonstrate how bioinformatics tools are used as a part of the research process. Currently, all Coffee Breaks are written by NCBI staff.[19] Each report is about 400 words and is usually based on a discovery reported in one or more articles from recently published, peer-reviewed literature.[20] This site has new articles every few weeks, so it can be considered an online magazine of sorts. It is intended for general background information. You can access the Coffee Break Web site at the following hyperlink: **http://www.ncbi.nlm.nih.gov/Coffeebreak/**.

Other Commercial Databases

In addition to resources maintained by official agencies, other databases exist that are commercial ventures addressing medical professionals. Here are some examples that may interest you:

- **CliniWeb International:** Index and table of contents to selected clinical information on the Internet; see **http://www.ohsu.edu/cliniweb/**.

- **Medical World Search:** Searches full text from thousands of selected medical sites on the Internet; see **http://www.mwsearch.com/**.

---

[18] Adapted from **http://www.ncbi.nlm.nih.gov/Coffeebreak/Archive/FAQ.html**.

[19] The figure that accompanies each article is frequently supplied by an expert external to NCBI, in which case the source of the figure is cited. The result is an interactive tutorial that tells a biological story.

[20] After a brief introduction that sets the work described into a broader context, the report focuses on how a molecular understanding can provide explanations of observed biology and lead to therapies for diseases. Each vignette is accompanied by a figure and hypertext links that lead to a series of pages that interactively show how NCBI tools and resources are used in the research process.

APPENDIX B. PATIENT RESOURCES

Overview

Official agencies, as well as federally funded institutions supported by national grants, frequently publish a variety of guidelines written with the patient in mind. These are typically called "Fact Sheets" or "Guidelines." They can take the form of a brochure, information kit, pamphlet, or flyer. Often they are only a few pages in length. Since new guidelines on osteopathy can appear at any moment and be published by a number of sources, the best approach to finding guidelines is to systematically scan the Internet-based services that post them.

Patient Guideline Sources

The remainder of this chapter directs you to sources which either publish or can help you find additional guidelines on topics related to osteopathy. Due to space limitations, these sources are listed in a concise manner. Do not hesitate to consult the following sources by either using the Internet hyperlink provided, or, in cases where the contact information is provided, contacting the publisher or author directly.

The National Institutes of Health

The NIH gateway to patients is located at **http://health.nih.gov/**. From this site, you can search across various sources and institutes, a number of which are summarized below.

Topic Pages: MEDLINEplus

The National Library of Medicine has created a vast and patient-oriented healthcare information portal called MEDLINEplus. Within this Internet-based system are "health topic pages" which list links to available materials relevant to osteopathy. To access this system, log on to **http://www.nlm.nih.gov/medlineplus/healthtopics.html**. From there you can either search using the alphabetical index or browse by broad topic areas. Recently, MEDLINEplus listed the following when searched for "osteopathy":

Bone Cancer
http://www.nlm.nih.gov/medlineplus/bonecancer.html

Bone Diseases
http://www.nlm.nih.gov/medlineplus/bonediseases.html

Osteogenesis Imperfecta
http://www.nlm.nih.gov/medlineplus/osteogenesisimperfecta.html

Osteoporosis
http://www.nlm.nih.gov/medlineplus/osteoporosis.html

Paget's Disease of Bone
http://www.nlm.nih.gov/medlineplus/pagetsdiseaseofbone.html

You may also choose to use the search utility provided by MEDLINEplus at the following Web address: **http://www.nlm.nih.gov/medlineplus/**. Simply type a keyword into the search box and click "Search." This utility is similar to the NIH search utility, with the exception that it only includes materials that are linked within the MEDLINEplus system (mostly patient-oriented information). It also has the disadvantage of generating unstructured results. We recommend, therefore, that you use this method only if you have a very targeted search.

The NIH Search Utility

The NIH search utility allows you to search for documents on over 100 selected Web sites that comprise the NIH-WEB-SPACE. Each of these servers is "crawled" and indexed on an ongoing basis. Your search will produce a list of various documents, all of which will relate in some way to osteopathy. The drawbacks of this approach are that the information is not organized by theme and that the references are often a mix of information for professionals and patients. Nevertheless, a large number of the listed Web sites provide useful background information. We can only recommend this route, therefore, for relatively rare or specific disorders, or when using highly targeted searches. To use the NIH search utility, visit the following Web page: **http://search.nih.gov/index.html**.

Additional Web Sources

A number of Web sites are available to the public that often link to government sites. These can also point you in the direction of essential information. The following is a representative sample:

- AOL: **http://search.aol.com/cat.adp?id=168&layer=&from=subcats**

- Family Village: **http://www.familyvillage.wisc.edu/specific.htm**

- Google: **http://directory.google.com/Top/Health/Conditions_and_Diseases/**

- Med Help International: **http://www.medhelp.org/HealthTopics/A.html**

- Open Directory Project: **http://dmoz.org/Health/Conditions_and_Diseases/**

- Yahoo.com: **http://dir.yahoo.com/Health/Diseases_and_Conditions/**

- WebMD®Health: **http://my.webmd.com/health_topics**

Finding Associations

There are several Internet directories that provide lists of medical associations with information on or resources relating to osteopathy. By consulting all of associations listed in this chapter, you will have nearly exhausted all sources for patient associations concerned with osteopathy.

The National Health Information Center (NHIC)

The National Health Information Center (NHIC) offers a free referral service to help people find organizations that provide information about osteopathy. For more information, see the NHIC's Web site at **http://www.health.gov/NHIC/** or contact an information specialist by calling 1-800-336-4797.

Directory of Health Organizations

The Directory of Health Organizations, provided by the National Library of Medicine Specialized Information Services, is a comprehensive source of information on associations. The Directory of Health Organizations database can be accessed via the Internet at **http://www.sis.nlm.nih.gov/Dir/DirMain.html**. It is composed of two parts: DIRLINE and Health Hotlines.

The DIRLINE database comprises some 10,000 records of organizations, research centers, and government institutes and associations that primarily focus on health and biomedicine. To access DIRLINE directly, go to the following Web site: **http://dirline.nlm.nih.gov/**. Simply type in "osteopathy" (or a synonym), and you will receive information on all relevant organizations listed in the database.

Health Hotlines directs you to toll-free numbers to over 300 organizations. You can access this database directly at **http://www.sis.nlm.nih.gov/hotlines/**. On this page, you are given the option to search by keyword or by browsing the subject list. When you have received your search results, click on the name of the organization for its description and contact information.

The Combined Health Information Database

Another comprehensive source of information on healthcare associations is the Combined Health Information Database. Using the "Detailed Search" option, you will need to limit your search to "Organizations" and "osteopathy". Type the following hyperlink into your Web browser: **http://chid.nih.gov/detail/detail.html**. To find associations, use the drop boxes at the bottom of the search page where "You may refine your search by." For publication date, select "All Years." Then, select your preferred language and the format option "Organization Resource Sheet." Type "osteopathy" (or synonyms) into the "For these words:" box. You should check back periodically with this database since it is updated every three months.

The National Organization for Rare Disorders, Inc.

The National Organization for Rare Disorders, Inc. has prepared a Web site that provides, at no charge, lists of associations organized by health topic. You can access this database at the following Web site: **http://www.rarediseases.org/search/orgsearch.html**. Type "osteopathy" (or a synonym) into the search box, and click "Submit Query."

APPENDIX C. FINDING MEDICAL LIBRARIES

Overview

In this Appendix, we show you how to quickly find a medical library in your area.

Preparation

Your local public library and medical libraries have interlibrary loan programs with the National Library of Medicine (NLM), one of the largest medical collections in the world. According to the NLM, most of the literature in the general and historical collections of the National Library of Medicine is available on interlibrary loan to any library. If you would like to access NLM medical literature, then visit a library in your area that can request the publications for you.[21]

Finding a Local Medical Library

The quickest method to locate medical libraries is to use the Internet-based directory published by the National Network of Libraries of Medicine (NN/LM). This network includes 4626 members and affiliates that provide many services to librarians, health professionals, and the public. To find a library in your area, simply visit **http://nnlm.gov/members/adv.html** or call 1-800-338-7657.

Medical Libraries in the U.S. and Canada

In addition to the NN/LM, the National Library of Medicine (NLM) lists a number of libraries with reference facilities that are open to the public. The following is the NLM's list and includes hyperlinks to each library's Web site. These Web pages can provide information on hours of operation and other restrictions. The list below is a small sample of

---

[21] Adapted from the NLM: **http://www.nlm.nih.gov/psd/cas/interlibrary.html**.

libraries recommended by the National Library of Medicine (sorted alphabetically by name of the U.S. state or Canadian province where the library is located)[22]:

- **Alabama:** Health InfoNet of Jefferson County (Jefferson County Library Cooperative, Lister Hill Library of the Health Sciences), **http://www.uab.edu/infonet/**

- **Alabama:** Richard M. Scrushy Library (American Sports Medicine Institute)

- **Arizona:** Samaritan Regional Medical Center: The Learning Center (Samaritan Health System, Phoenix, Arizona), **http://www.samaritan.edu/library/bannerlibs.htm**

- **California:** Kris Kelly Health Information Center (St. Joseph Health System, Humboldt), **http://www.humboldt1.com/~kkhic/index.html**

- **California:** Community Health Library of Los Gatos, **http://www.healthlib.org/orgresources.html**

- **California:** Consumer Health Program and Services (CHIPS) (County of Los Angeles Public Library, Los Angeles County Harbor-UCLA Medical Center Library) - Carson, CA, **http://www.colapublib.org/services/chips.html**

- **California:** Gateway Health Library (Sutter Gould Medical Foundation)

- **California:** Health Library (Stanford University Medical Center), **http://www-med.stanford.edu/healthlibrary/**

- **California:** Patient Education Resource Center - Health Information and Resources (University of California, San Francisco), **http://sfghdean.ucsf.edu/barnett/PERC/default.asp**

- **California:** Redwood Health Library (Petaluma Health Care District), **http://www.phcd.org/rdwdlib.html**

- **California:** Los Gatos PlaneTree Health Library, **http://planetreesanjose.org/**

- **California:** Sutter Resource Library (Sutter Hospitals Foundation, Sacramento), **http://suttermedicalcenter.org/library/**

- **California:** Health Sciences Libraries (University of California, Davis), **http://www.lib.ucdavis.edu/healthsci/**

- **California:** ValleyCare Health Library & Ryan Comer Cancer Resource Center (ValleyCare Health System, Pleasanton), **http://gaelnet.stmarys-ca.edu/other.libs/gbal/east/vchl.html**

- **California:** Washington Community Health Resource Library (Fremont), **http://www.healthlibrary.org/**

- **Colorado:** William V. Gervasini Memorial Library (Exempla Healthcare), **http://www.saintjosephdenver.org/yourhealth/libraries/**

- **Connecticut:** Hartford Hospital Health Science Libraries (Hartford Hospital), **http://www.harthosp.org/library/**

- **Connecticut:** Healthnet: Connecticut Consumer Health Information Center (University of Connecticut Health Center, Lyman Maynard Stowe Library), **http://library.uchc.edu/departm/hnet/**

---

[22] Abstracted from **http://www.nlm.nih.gov/medlineplus/libraries.html**.

- **Connecticut:** Waterbury Hospital Health Center Library (Waterbury Hospital, Waterbury), **http://www.waterburyhospital.com/library/consumer.shtml**

- **Delaware:** Consumer Health Library (Christiana Care Health System, Eugene du Pont Preventive Medicine & Rehabilitation Institute, Wilmington), **http://www.christianacare.org/health_guide/health_guide_pmri_health_info.cfm**

- **Delaware:** Lewis B. Flinn Library (Delaware Academy of Medicine, Wilmington), **http://www.delamed.org/chls.html**

- **Georgia:** Family Resource Library (Medical College of Georgia, Augusta), **http://cmc.mcg.edu/kids_families/fam_resources/fam_res_lib/frl.htm**

- **Georgia:** Health Resource Center (Medical Center of Central Georgia, Macon), **http://www.mccg.org/hrc/hrchome.asp**

- **Hawaii:** Hawaii Medical Library: Consumer Health Information Service (Hawaii Medical Library, Honolulu), **http://hml.org/CHIS/**

- **Idaho:** DeArmond Consumer Health Library (Kootenai Medical Center, Coeur d'Alene), **http://www.nicon.org/DeArmond/index.htm**

- **Illinois:** Health Learning Center of Northwestern Memorial Hospital (Chicago), **http://www.nmh.org/health_info/hlc.html**

- **Illinois:** Medical Library (OSF Saint Francis Medical Center, Peoria), **http://www.osfsaintfrancis.org/general/library/**

- **Kentucky:** Medical Library - Services for Patients, Families, Students & the Public (Central Baptist Hospital, Lexington), **http://www.centralbap.com/education/community/library.cfm**

- **Kentucky:** University of Kentucky - Health Information Library (Chandler Medical Center, Lexington), **http://www.mc.uky.edu/PatientEd/**

- **Louisiana:** Alton Ochsner Medical Foundation Library (Alton Ochsner Medical Foundation, New Orleans), **http://www.ochsner.org/library/**

- **Louisiana:** Louisiana State University Health Sciences Center Medical Library-Shreveport, **http://lib-sh.lsuhsc.edu/**

- **Maine:** Franklin Memorial Hospital Medical Library (Franklin Memorial Hospital, Farmington), **http://www.fchn.org/fmh/lib.htm**

- **Maine:** Gerrish-True Health Sciences Library (Central Maine Medical Center, Lewiston), **http://www.cmmc.org/library/library.html**

- **Maine:** Hadley Parrot Health Science Library (Eastern Maine Healthcare, Bangor), **http://www.emh.org/hll/hpl/guide.htm**

- **Maine:** Maine Medical Center Library (Maine Medical Center, Portland), **http://www.mmc.org/library/**

- **Maine:** Parkview Hospital (Brunswick), **http://www.parkviewhospital.org/**

- **Maine:** Southern Maine Medical Center Health Sciences Library (Southern Maine Medical Center, Biddeford), **http://www.smmc.org/services/service.php3?choice=10**

- **Maine:** Stephens Memorial Hospital's Health Information Library (Western Maine Health, Norway), **http://www.wmhcc.org/Library/**

- **Manitoba, Canada:** Consumer & Patient Health Information Service (University of Manitoba Libraries), http://www.umanitoba.ca/libraries/units/health/reference/chis.html

- **Manitoba, Canada:** J.W. Crane Memorial Library (Deer Lodge Centre, Winnipeg), http://www.deerlodge.mb.ca/crane_library/about.asp

- **Maryland:** Health Information Center at the Wheaton Regional Library (Montgomery County, Dept. of Public Libraries, Wheaton Regional Library), http://www.mont.lib.md.us/healthinfo/hic.asp

- **Massachusetts:** Baystate Medical Center Library (Baystate Health System), http://www.baystatehealth.com/1024/

- **Massachusetts:** Boston University Medical Center Alumni Medical Library (Boston University Medical Center), http://med-libwww.bu.edu/library/lib.html

- **Massachusetts:** Lowell General Hospital Health Sciences Library (Lowell General Hospital, Lowell), http://www.lowellgeneral.org/library/HomePageLinks/WWW.htm

- **Massachusetts:** Paul E. Woodard Health Sciences Library (New England Baptist Hospital, Boston), http://www.nebh.org/health_lib.asp

- **Massachusetts:** St. Luke's Hospital Health Sciences Library (St. Luke's Hospital, Southcoast Health System, New Bedford), http://www.southcoast.org/library/

- **Massachusetts:** Treadwell Library Consumer Health Reference Center (Massachusetts General Hospital), http://www.mgh.harvard.edu/library/chrcindex.html

- **Massachusetts:** UMass HealthNet (University of Massachusetts Medical School, Worchester), http://healthnet.umassmed.edu/

- **Michigan:** Botsford General Hospital Library - Consumer Health (Botsford General Hospital, Library & Internet Services), http://www.botsfordlibrary.org/consumer.htm

- **Michigan:** Helen DeRoy Medical Library (Providence Hospital and Medical Centers), http://www.providence-hospital.org/library/

- **Michigan:** Marquette General Hospital - Consumer Health Library (Marquette General Hospital, Health Information Center), http://www.mgh.org/center.html

- **Michigan:** Patient Education Resouce Center - University of Michigan Cancer Center (University of Michigan Comprehensive Cancer Center, Ann Arbor), http://www.cancer.med.umich.edu/learn/leares.htm

- **Michigan:** Sladen Library & Center for Health Information Resources - Consumer Health Information (Detroit), http://www.henryford.com/body.cfm?id=39330

- **Montana:** Center for Health Information (St. Patrick Hospital and Health Sciences Center, Missoula)

- **National:** Consumer Health Library Directory (Medical Library Association, Consumer and Patient Health Information Section), http://caphis.mlanet.org/directory/index.html

- **National:** National Network of Libraries of Medicine (National Library of Medicine) - provides library services for health professionals in the United States who do not have access to a medical library, http://nnlm.gov/

- **National:** NN/LM List of Libraries Serving the Public (National Network of Libraries of Medicine), http://nnlm.gov/members/

- **Nevada:** Health Science Library, West Charleston Library (Las Vegas-Clark County Library District, Las Vegas), **http://www.lvccld.org/special_collections/medical/index.htm**

- **New Hampshire:** Dartmouth Biomedical Libraries (Dartmouth College Library, Hanover), **http://www.dartmouth.edu/~biomed/resources.htmld/conshealth.htmld/**

- **New Jersey:** Consumer Health Library (Rahway Hospital, Rahway), **http://www.rahwayhospital.com/library.htm**

- **New Jersey:** Dr. Walter Phillips Health Sciences Library (Englewood Hospital and Medical Center, Englewood), **http://www.englewoodhospital.com/links/index.htm**

- **New Jersey:** Meland Foundation (Englewood Hospital and Medical Center, Englewood), **http://www.geocities.com/ResearchTriangle/9360/**

- **New York:** Choices in Health Information (New York Public Library) - NLM Consumer Pilot Project participant, **http://www.nypl.org/branch/health/links.html**

- **New York:** Health Information Center (Upstate Medical University, State University of New York, Syracuse), **http://www.upstate.edu/library/hic/**

- **New York:** Health Sciences Library (Long Island Jewish Medical Center, New Hyde Park), **http://www.lij.edu/library/library.html**

- **New York:** ViaHealth Medical Library (Rochester General Hospital), **http://www.nyam.org/library/**

- **Ohio:** Consumer Health Library (Akron General Medical Center, Medical & Consumer Health Library), **http://www.akrongeneral.org/hwlibrary.htm**

- **Oklahoma:** The Health Information Center at Saint Francis Hospital (Saint Francis Health System, Tulsa), **http://www.sfh-tulsa.com/services/healthinfo.asp**

- **Oregon:** Planetree Health Resource Center (Mid-Columbia Medical Center, The Dalles), **http://www.mcmc.net/phrc/**

- **Pennsylvania:** Community Health Information Library (Milton S. Hershey Medical Center, Hershey), **http://www.hmc.psu.edu/commhealth/**

- **Pennsylvania:** Community Health Resource Library (Geisinger Medical Center, Danville), **http://www.geisinger.edu/education/commlib.shtml**

- **Pennsylvania:** HealthInfo Library (Moses Taylor Hospital, Scranton), **http://www.mth.org/healthwellness.html**

- **Pennsylvania:** Hopwood Library (University of Pittsburgh, Health Sciences Library System, Pittsburgh), **http://www.hsls.pitt.edu/guides/chi/hopwood/index_html**

- **Pennsylvania:** Koop Community Health Information Center (College of Physicians of Philadelphia), **http://www.collphyphil.org/kooppg1.shtml**

- **Pennsylvania:** Learning Resources Center - Medical Library (Susquehanna Health System, Williamsport), **http://www.shscares.org/services/lrc/index.asp**

- **Pennsylvania:** Medical Library (UPMC Health System, Pittsburgh), **http://www.upmc.edu/passavant/library.htm**

- **Quebec, Canada:** Medical Library (Montreal General Hospital), **http://www.mghlib.mcgill.ca/**

- **South Dakota:** Rapid City Regional Hospital Medical Library (Rapid City Regional Hospital), **http://www.rcrh.org/Services/Library/Default.asp**

- **Texas:** Houston HealthWays (Houston Academy of Medicine-Texas Medical Center Library), **http://hhw.library.tmc.edu/**

- **Washington:** Community Health Library (Kittitas Valley Community Hospital), **http://www.kvch.com/**

- **Washington:** Southwest Washington Medical Center Library (Southwest Washington Medical Center, Vancouver), **http://www.swmedicalcenter.com/body.cfm?id=72**

ONLINE GLOSSARIES

The Internet provides access to a number of free-to-use medical dictionaries. The National Library of Medicine has compiled the following list of online dictionaries:

- ADAM Medical Encyclopedia (A.D.A.M., Inc.), comprehensive medical reference: **http://www.nlm.nih.gov/medlineplus/encyclopedia.html**

- MedicineNet.com Medical Dictionary (MedicineNet, Inc.): **http://www.medterms.com/Script/Main/hp.asp**

- Merriam-Webster Medical Dictionary (Inteli-Health, Inc.): **http://www.intelihealth.com/IH/**

- Multilingual Glossary of Technical and Popular Medical Terms in Eight European Languages (European Commission) - Danish, Dutch, English, French, German, Italian, Portuguese, and Spanish: **http://allserv.rug.ac.be/~rvdstich/eugloss/welcome.html**

- On-line Medical Dictionary (CancerWEB): **http://cancerweb.ncl.ac.uk/omd/**

- Rare Diseases Terms (Office of Rare Diseases): **http://ord.aspensys.com/asp/diseases/diseases.asp**

- Technology Glossary (National Library of Medicine) - Health Care Technology: **http://www.nlm.nih.gov/nichsr/ta101/ta10108.htm**

Beyond these, MEDLINEplus contains a very patient-friendly encyclopedia covering every aspect of medicine (licensed from A.D.A.M., Inc.). The ADAM Medical Encyclopedia can be accessed at **http://www.nlm.nih.gov/medlineplus/encyclopedia.html**. ADAM is also available on commercial Web sites such as drkoop.com (**http://www.drkoop.com/**) and Web MD (**http://my.webmd.com/adam/asset/adam_disease_articles/a_to_z/a**).

Online Dictionary Directories

The following are additional online directories compiled by the National Library of Medicine, including a number of specialized medical dictionaries:

- Medical Dictionaries: Medical & Biological (World Health Organization): **http://www.who.int/hlt/virtuallibrary/English/diction.htm#Medical**

- MEL-Michigan Electronic Library List of Online Health and Medical Dictionaries (Michigan Electronic Library): **http://mel.lib.mi.us/health/health-dictionaries.html**

- Patient Education: Glossaries (DMOZ Open Directory Project): **http://dmoz.org/Health/Education/Patient_Education/Glossaries/**

- Web of Online Dictionaries (Bucknell University): **http://www.yourdictionary.com/diction5.html#medicine**

OSTEOPATHY DICTIONARY

The definitions below are derived from official public sources, including the National Institutes of Health [NIH] and the European Union [EU].

Abdominal: Having to do with the abdomen, which is the part of the body between the chest and the hips that contains the pancreas, stomach, intestines, liver, gallbladder, and other organs. [NIH]

Algorithms: A procedure consisting of a sequence of algebraic formulas and/or logical steps to calculate or determine a given task. [NIH]

Alkaline: Having the reactions of an alkali. [EU]

Alpha Particles: Positively charged particles composed of two protons and two neutrons, i.e., helium nuclei, emitted during disintegration of very heavy isotopes; a beam of alpha particles or an alpha ray has very strong ionizing power, but weak penetrability. [NIH]

Alternative medicine: Practices not generally recognized by the medical community as standard or conventional medical approaches and used instead of standard treatments. Alternative medicine includes the taking of dietary supplements, megadose vitamins, and herbal preparations; the drinking of special teas; and practices such as massage therapy, magnet therapy, spiritual healing, and meditation. [NIH]

Aluminum: A metallic element that has the atomic number 13, atomic symbol Al, and atomic weight 26.98. [NIH]

Amino acid: Any organic compound containing an amino (-NH2 and a carboxyl (- COOH) group. The 20 a-amino acids listed in the accompanying table are the amino acids from which proteins are synthesized by formation of peptide bonds during ribosomal translation of messenger RNA; all except glycine, which is not optically active, have the L configuration. Other amino acids occurring in proteins, such as hydroxyproline in collagen, are formed by posttranslational enzymatic modification of amino acids residues in polypeptide chains. There are also several important amino acids, such as the neurotransmitter y-aminobutyric acid, that have no relation to proteins. Abbreviated AA. [EU]

Amino Acid Sequence: The order of amino acids as they occur in a polypeptide chain. This is referred to as the primary structure of proteins. It is of fundamental importance in determining protein conformation. [NIH]

Amyloid: A general term for a variety of different proteins that accumulate as extracellular fibrils of 7-10 nm and have common structural features, including a beta-pleated sheet conformation and the ability to bind such dyes as Congo red and thioflavine (Kandel, Schwartz, and Jessel, Principles of Neural Science, 3rd ed). [NIH]

Anaemia: A reduction below normal in the number of erythrocytes per cu. mm., in the quantity of haemoglobin, or in the volume of packed red cells per 100 ml. of blood which occurs when the equilibrium between blood loss (through bleeding or destruction) and blood production is disturbed. [EU]

Anemia: A reduction in the number of circulating erythrocytes or in the quantity of hemoglobin. [NIH]

Ankle: That part of the lower limb directly above the foot. [NIH]

Anomalies: Birth defects; abnormalities. [NIH]

Anorexia: Lack or loss of appetite for food. Appetite is psychologic, dependent on memory and associations. Anorexia can be brought about by unattractive food, surroundings, or company. [NIH]

Anticonvulsant: An agent that prevents or relieves convulsions. [EU]

Antimetabolite: A chemical that is very similar to one required in a normal biochemical reaction in cells. Antimetabolites can stop or slow down the reaction. [NIH]

Antineoplastic: Inhibiting or preventing the development of neoplasms, checking the maturation and proliferation of malignant cells. [EU]

Aorta: The main trunk of the systemic arteries. [NIH]

Arteries: The vessels carrying blood away from the heart. [NIH]

Arthropathy: Any joint disease. [EU]

Articular: Of or pertaining to a joint. [EU]

Autopsy: Postmortem examination of the body. [NIH]

Back Pain: Acute or chronic pain located in the posterior regions of the trunk, including the thoracic, lumbar, sacral, or adjacent regions. [NIH]

Beta-pleated: Particular three-dimensional pattern of amyloidoses. [NIH]

Bewilderment: Impairment or loss of will power. [NIH]

Bile: An emulsifying agent produced in the liver and secreted into the duodenum. Its composition includes bile acids and salts, cholesterol, and electrolytes. It aids digestion of fats in the duodenum. [NIH]

Biotechnology: Body of knowledge related to the use of organisms, cells or cell-derived constituents for the purpose of developing products which are technically, scientifically and clinically useful. Alteration of biologic function at the molecular level (i.e., genetic engineering) is a central focus; laboratory methods used include transfection and cloning technologies, sequence and structure analysis algorithms, computer databases, and gene and protein structure function analysis and prediction. [NIH]

Blood Coagulation: The process of the interaction of blood coagulation factors that results in an insoluble fibrin clot. [NIH]

Blood pressure: The pressure of blood against the walls of a blood vessel or heart chamber. Unless there is reference to another location, such as the pulmonary artery or one of the heart chambers, it refers to the pressure in the systemic arteries, as measured, for example, in the forearm. [NIH]

Blood vessel: A tube in the body through which blood circulates. Blood vessels include a network of arteries, arterioles, capillaries, venules, and veins. [NIH]

Bone Resorption: Bone loss due to osteoclastic activity. [NIH]

Cadmium: An element with atomic symbol Cd, atomic number 48, and atomic weight 114. It is a metal and ingestion will lead to cadmium poisoning. [NIH]

Cadmium Poisoning: Poisoning occurring after exposure to cadmium compounds or fumes. It may cause gastrointestinal syndromes, anemia, or pneumonitis. [NIH]

Calcitonin: A peptide hormone that lowers calcium concentration in the blood. In humans, it is released by thyroid cells and acts to decrease the formation and absorptive activity of osteoclasts. Its role in regulating plasma calcium is much greater in children and in certain diseases than in normal adults. [NIH]

Calcium: A basic element found in nearly all organized tissues. It is a member of the alkaline earth family of metals with the atomic symbol Ca, atomic number 20, and atomic weight 40. Calcium is the most abundant mineral in the body and combines with phosphorus to form calcium phosphate in the bones and teeth. It is essential for the normal functioning of nerves and muscles and plays a role in blood coagulation (as factor IV) and in many enzymatic processes. [NIH]

Calcium Oxalate: The calcium salt of oxalic acid, occurring in the urine as crystals and in certain calculi. [NIH]

Cardiac: Having to do with the heart. [NIH]

Cardiovascular: Having to do with the heart and blood vessels. [NIH]

Cardiovascular disease: Any abnormal condition characterized by dysfunction of the heart and blood vessels. CVD includes atherosclerosis (especially coronary heart disease, which can lead to heart attacks), cerebrovascular disease (e.g., stroke), and hypertension (high blood pressure). [NIH]

Cell: The individual unit that makes up all of the tissues of the body. All living things are made up of one or more cells. [NIH]

Cell Division: The fission of a cell. [NIH]

Cell proliferation: An increase in the number of cells as a result of cell growth and cell division. [NIH]

Central Nervous System: The main information-processing organs of the nervous system, consisting of the brain, spinal cord, and meninges. [NIH]

Cerebrovascular: Pertaining to the blood vessels of the cerebrum, or brain. [EU]

Chiropractic: A system of treating bodily disorders by manipulation of the spine and other parts, based on the belief that the cause is the abnormal functioning of a nerve. [NIH]

Chronic: A disease or condition that persists or progresses over a long period of time. [NIH]

Clinical trial: A research study that tests how well new medical treatments or other interventions work in people. Each study is designed to test new methods of screening, prevention, diagnosis, or treatment of a disease. [NIH]

Cloning: The production of a number of genetically identical individuals; in genetic engineering, a process for the efficient replication of a great number of identical DNA molecules. [NIH]

Cognitive restructuring: A method of identifying and replacing fear-promoting, irrational beliefs with more realistic and functional ones. [NIH]

Collagen: A polypeptide substance comprising about one third of the total protein in mammalian organisms. It is the main constituent of skin, connective tissue, and the organic substance of bones and teeth. Different forms of collagen are produced in the body but all consist of three alpha-polypeptide chains arranged in a triple helix. Collagen is differentiated from other fibrous proteins, such as elastin, by the content of proline, hydroxyproline, and hydroxylysine; by the absence of tryptophan; and particularly by the high content of polar groups which are responsible for its swelling properties. [NIH]

Complement: A term originally used to refer to the heat-labile factor in serum that causes immune cytolysis, the lysis of antibody-coated cells, and now referring to the entire functionally related system comprising at least 20 distinct serum proteins that is the effector not only of immune cytolysis but also of other biologic functions. Complement activation occurs by two different sequences, the classic and alternative pathways. The proteins of the classic pathway are termed 'components of complement' and are designated by the symbols C1 through C9. C1 is a calcium-dependent complex of three distinct proteins C1q, C1r and C1s. The proteins of the alternative pathway (collectively referred to as the properdin system) and complement regulatory proteins are known by semisystematic or trivial names.

Fragments resulting from proteolytic cleavage of complement proteins are designated with lower-case letter suffixes, e.g., C3a. Inactivated fragments may be designated with the suffix 'i', e.g. C3bi. Activated components or complexes with biological activity are designated by a bar over the symbol e.g. C1 or C4b,2a. The classic pathway is activated by the binding of C1 to classic pathway activators, primarily antigen-antibody complexes containing IgM, IgG1, IgG3; C1q binds to a single IgM molecule or two adjacent IgG molecules. The alternative pathway can be activated by IgA immune complexes and also by nonimmunologic materials including bacterial endotoxins, microbial polysaccharides, and cell walls. Activation of the classic pathway triggers an enzymatic cascade involving C1, C4, C2 and C3; activation of the alternative pathway triggers a cascade involving C3 and factors B, D and P. Both result in the cleavage of C5 and the formation of the membrane attack complex. Complement activation also results in the formation of many biologically active complement fragments that act as anaphylatoxins, opsonins, or chemotactic factors. [EU]

Complementary and alternative medicine: CAM. Forms of treatment that are used in addition to (complementary) or instead of (alternative) standard treatments. These practices are not considered standard medical approaches. CAM includes dietary supplements, megadose vitamins, herbal preparations, special teas, massage therapy, magnet therapy, spiritual healing, and meditation. [NIH]

Complementary medicine: Practices not generally recognized by the medical community as standard or conventional medical approaches and used to enhance or complement the standard treatments. Complementary medicine includes the taking of dietary supplements, megadose vitamins, and herbal preparations; the drinking of special teas; and practices such as massage therapy, magnet therapy, spiritual healing, and meditation. [NIH]

Computational Biology: A field of biology concerned with the development of techniques for the collection and manipulation of biological data, and the use of such data to make biological discoveries or predictions. This field encompasses all computational methods and theories applicable to molecular biology and areas of computer-based techniques for solving biological problems including manipulation of models and datasets. [NIH]

Confusion: A mental state characterized by bewilderment, emotional disturbance, lack of clear thinking, and perceptual disorientation. [NIH]

Consciousness: Sense of awareness of self and of the environment. [NIH]

Contraindications: Any factor or sign that it is unwise to pursue a certain kind of action or treatment, e. g. giving a general anesthetic to a person with pneumonia. [NIH]

Convulsions: A general term referring to sudden and often violent motor activity of cerebral or brainstem origin. Convulsions may also occur in the absence of an electrical cerebral discharge (e.g., in response to hypotension). [NIH]

Coronary: Encircling in the manner of a crown; a term applied to vessels; nerves, ligaments, etc. The term usually denotes the arteries that supply the heart muscle and, by extension, a pathologic involvement of them. [EU]

Coronary heart disease: A type of heart disease caused by narrowing of the coronary arteries that feed the heart, which needs a constant supply of oxygen and nutrients carried by the blood in the coronary arteries. When the coronary arteries become narrowed or clogged by fat and cholesterol deposits and cannot supply enough blood to the heart, CHD results. [NIH]

Coronary Thrombosis: Presence of a thrombus in a coronary artery, often causing a myocardial infarction. [NIH]

Cortex: The outer layer of an organ or other body structure, as distinguished from the internal substance. [EU]

Cortical: Pertaining to or of the nature of a cortex or bark. [EU]

Cranial: Pertaining to the cranium, or to the anterior (in animals) or superior (in humans) end of the body. [EU]

Dehydration: The condition that results from excessive loss of body water. [NIH]

Dementia: An acquired organic mental disorder with loss of intellectual abilities of sufficient severity to interfere with social or occupational functioning. The dysfunction is multifaceted and involves memory, behavior, personality, judgment, attention, spatial relations, language, abstract thought, and other executive functions. The intellectual decline is usually progressive, and initially spares the level of consciousness. [NIH]

Dermis: A layer of vascular connective tissue underneath the epidermis. The surface of the dermis contains sensitive papillae. Embedded in or beneath the dermis are sweat glands, hair follicles, and sebaceous glands. [NIH]

Diabetes Mellitus: A heterogeneous group of disorders that share glucose intolerance in common. [NIH]

Diagnostic procedure: A method used to identify a disease. [NIH]

Dialyzer: A part of the hemodialysis machine. (See hemodialysis under dialysis.) The dialyzer has two sections separated by a membrane. One section holds dialysate. The other holds the patient's blood. [NIH]

Diffusion: The tendency of a gas or solute to pass from a point of higher pressure or concentration to a point of lower pressure or concentration and to distribute itself throughout the available space; a major mechanism of biological transport. [NIH]

Digestion: The process of breakdown of food for metabolism and use by the body. [NIH]

Direct: 1. Straight; in a straight line. 2. Performed immediately and without the intervention of subsidiary means. [EU]

Disorientation: The loss of proper bearings, or a state of mental confusion as to time, place, or identity. [EU]

Distemper: A name for several highly contagious viral diseases of animals, especially canine distemper. In dogs, it is caused by the canine distemper virus (distemper virus, canine). It is characterized by a diphasic fever, leukopenia, gastrointestinal and respiratory inflammation and sometimes, neurologic complications. In cats it is known as feline panleukopenia. [NIH]

Distemper Virus, Canine: A species of morbillivirus causing distemper in dogs, wolves, foxes, raccoons, and ferrets. [NIH]

Dominance: In genetics, the full phenotypic expression of a gene in both heterozygotes and homozygotes. [EU]

Drive: A state of internal activity of an organism that is a necessary condition before a given stimulus will elicit a class of responses; e.g., a certain level of hunger (drive) must be present before food will elicit an eating response. [NIH]

Ductus Arteriosus: A fetal blood vessel connecting the pulmonary artery with the descending aorta. [NIH]

Dyes: Chemical substances that are used to stain and color other materials. The coloring may or may not be permanent. Dyes can also be used as therapeutic agents and test reagents in medicine and scientific research. [NIH]

Efficacy: The extent to which a specific intervention, procedure, regimen, or service produces a beneficial result under ideal conditions. Ideally, the determination of efficacy is based on the results of a randomized control trial. [NIH]

Electrolyte: A substance that dissociates into ions when fused or in solution, and thus becomes capable of conducting electricity; an ionic solute. [EU]

Electrons: Stable elementary particles having the smallest known negative charge, present in all elements; also called negatrons. Positively charged electrons are called positrons. The numbers, energies and arrangement of electrons around atomic nuclei determine the chemical identities of elements. Beams of electrons are called cathode rays or beta rays, the latter being a high-energy biproduct of nuclear decay. [NIH]

Endotoxins: Toxins closely associated with the living cytoplasm or cell wall of certain microorganisms, which do not readily diffuse into the culture medium, but are released upon lysis of the cells. [NIH]

Environmental Health: The science of controlling or modifying those conditions, influences, or forces surrounding man which relate to promoting, establishing, and maintaining health. [NIH]

Enzymatic: Phase where enzyme cuts the precursor protein. [NIH]

Enzyme: A protein that speeds up chemical reactions in the body. [NIH]

Epigastric: Having to do with the upper middle area of the abdomen. [NIH]

Erythrocytes: Red blood cells. Mature erythrocytes are non-nucleated, biconcave disks containing hemoglobin whose function is to transport oxygen. [NIH]

Exocrine: Secreting outwardly, via a duct. [EU]

Exostoses: Benign hypertrophy that projects outward from the surface of bone, often containing a cartilaginous component. [NIH]

Extensor: A muscle whose contraction tends to straighten a limb; the antagonist of a flexor. [NIH]

Extracellular: Outside a cell or cells. [EU]

Extracellular Matrix: A meshwork-like substance found within the extracellular space and in association with the basement membrane of the cell surface. It promotes cellular proliferation and provides a supporting structure to which cells or cell lysates in culture dishes adhere. [NIH]

Family Planning: Programs or services designed to assist the family in controlling reproduction by either improving or diminishing fertility. [NIH]

Fat: Total lipids including phospholipids. [NIH]

Feline Panleukopenia: A highly contagious DNA virus infection of the cat family and of mink, characterized by fever, enteritis and bone marrow changes. It is also called feline ataxia, feline agranulocytosis, feline infectious enteritis, cat fever, cat plague, show fever. [NIH]

Femoral: Pertaining to the femur, or to the thigh. [EU]

Femur: The longest and largest bone of the skeleton, it is situated between the hip and the knee. [NIH]

Fetal Blood: Blood of the fetus. Exchange of nutrients and waste between the fetal and maternal blood occurs via the placenta. The cord blood is blood contained in the umbilical vessels at the time of delivery. [NIH]

Focal Dermal Hypoplasia: A genetic skin disease characterized by hypoplasia of the dermis, herniations of fat, and hand anomalies. It is found exclusively in females and transmitted as an X-linked dominant trait. [NIH]

Gastrectomy: An operation to remove all or part of the stomach. [NIH]

Gastrin: A hormone released after eating. Gastrin causes the stomach to produce more acid. [NIH]

Gastrointestinal: Refers to the stomach and intestines. [NIH]

Gene: The functional and physical unit of heredity passed from parent to offspring. Genes are pieces of DNA, and most genes contain the information for making a specific protein. [NIH]

Genetics: The biological science that deals with the phenomena and mechanisms of heredity. [NIH]

Geriatric: Pertaining to the treatment of the aged. [EU]

Gland: An organ that produces and releases one or more substances for use in the body. Some glands produce fluids that affect tissues or organs. Others produce hormones or participate in blood production. [NIH]

Glomerular: Pertaining to or of the nature of a glomerulus, especially a renal glomerulus. [EU]

Glucose: D-Glucose. A primary source of energy for living organisms. It is naturally occurring and is found in fruits and other parts of plants in its free state. It is used therapeutically in fluid and nutrient replacement. [NIH]

Glucose Intolerance: A pathological state in which the fasting plasma glucose level is less than 140 mg per deciliter and the 30-, 60-, or 90-minute plasma glucose concentration following a glucose tolerance test exceeds 200 mg per deciliter. This condition is seen frequently in diabetes mellitus but also occurs with other diseases. [NIH]

Glycine: A non-essential amino acid. It is found primarily in gelatin and silk fibroin and used therapeutically as a nutrient. It is also a fast inhibitory neurotransmitter. [NIH]

Governing Board: The group in which legal authority is vested for the control of health-related institutions and organizations. [NIH]

Haemodialysis: The removal of certain elements from the blood by virtue of the difference in the rates of their diffusion through a semipermeable membrane, e.g., by means of a haemodialyzer. [EU]

Health Services: Services for the diagnosis and treatment of disease and the maintenance of health. [NIH]

Heart attack: A seizure of weak or abnormal functioning of the heart. [NIH]

Hemodialysis: The use of a machine to clean wastes from the blood after the kidneys have failed. The blood travels through tubes to a dialyzer, which removes wastes and extra fluid. The cleaned blood then flows through another set of tubes back into the body. [NIH]

Hemofiltration: Extracorporeal ultrafiltration technique without hemodialysis for treatment of fluid overload and electrolyte disturbances affecting renal, cardiac, or pulmonary function. [NIH]

Hepatic: Refers to the liver. [NIH]

Heredity: 1. The genetic transmission of a particular quality or trait from parent to offspring. 2. The genetic constitution of an individual. [EU]

Heterozygotes: Having unlike alleles at one or more corresponding loci on homologous chromosomes. [NIH]

Histology: The study of tissues and cells under a microscope. [NIH]

Homozygotes: An individual having a homozygous gene pair. [NIH]

Hormone: A substance in the body that regulates certain organs. Hormones such as gastrin help in breaking down food. Some hormones come from cells in the stomach and small intestine. [NIH]

Hydroxyproline: A hydroxylated form of the imino acid proline. A deficiency in ascorbic acid can result in impaired hydroxyproline formation. [NIH]

Hyperostosis: Increase in the mass of bone per unit volume. [NIH]

Hyperoxaluria: Excretion of an excessive amount of oxalate in the urine. [NIH]

Hypersensitivity: Altered reactivity to an antigen, which can result in pathologic reactions upon subsequent exposure to that particular antigen. [NIH]

Hypertension: Persistently high arterial blood pressure. Currently accepted threshold levels are 140 mm Hg systolic and 90 mm Hg diastolic pressure. [NIH]

Hyperthyroidism: Excessive functional activity of the thyroid gland. [NIH]

Hypertrophy: General increase in bulk of a part or organ, not due to tumor formation, nor to an increase in the number of cells. [NIH]

Hypoplasia: Incomplete development or underdevelopment of an organ or tissue. [EU]

Idiopathic: Describes a disease of unknown cause. [NIH]

Idiosyncrasy: An abnormal susceptibility to some drug, protein, or other agent which is peculiar to the individual. [EU]

Immune response: The activity of the immune system against foreign substances (antigens). [NIH]

Immunosuppressant: An agent capable of suppressing immune responses. [EU]

In vitro: In the laboratory (outside the body). The opposite of in vivo (in the body). [NIH]

In vivo: In the body. The opposite of in vitro (outside the body or in the laboratory). [NIH]

Infarction: A pathological process consisting of a sudden insufficient blood supply to an area, which results in necrosis of that area. It is usually caused by a thrombus, an embolus, or a vascular torsion. [NIH]

Infection: 1. Invasion and multiplication of microorganisms in body tissues, which may be clinically unapparent or result in local cellular injury due to competitive metabolism, toxins, intracellular replication, or antigen-antibody response. The infection may remain localized, subclinical, and temporary if the body's defensive mechanisms are effective. A local infection may persist and spread by extension to become an acute, subacute, or chronic clinical infection or disease state. A local infection may also become systemic when the microorganisms gain access to the lymphatic or vascular system. 2. An infectious disease. [EU]

Inflammation: A pathological process characterized by injury or destruction of tissues caused by a variety of cytologic and chemical reactions. It is usually manifested by typical signs of pain, heat, redness, swelling, and loss of function. [NIH]

Ingestion: Taking into the body by mouth [NIH]

Insulin: A protein hormone secreted by beta cells of the pancreas. Insulin plays a major role in the regulation of glucose metabolism, generally promoting the cellular utilization of glucose. It is also an important regulator of protein and lipid metabolism. Insulin is used as a drug to control insulin-dependent diabetes mellitus. [NIH]

Interstitial: Pertaining to or situated between parts or in the interspaces of a tissue. [EU]

Intestinal: Having to do with the intestines. [NIH]

Intestines: The section of the alimentary canal from the stomach to the anus. It includes the large intestine and small intestine. [NIH]

Intoxication: Poisoning, the state of being poisoned. [EU]

Isoenzyme: Different forms of an enzyme, usually occurring in different tissues. The isoenzymes of a particular enzyme catalyze the same reaction but they differ in some of their properties. [NIH]

Kb: A measure of the length of DNA fragments, 1 Kb = 1000 base pairs. The largest DNA fragments are up to 50 kilobases long. [NIH]

Keto: It consists of 8 carbon atoms and within the endotoxins, it connects poysaccharide and lipid A. [NIH]

Kidney stone: A stone that develops from crystals that form in urine and build up on the inner surfaces of the kidney, in the renal pelvis, or in the ureters. [NIH]

Kidney Transplantation: The transference of a kidney from one human or animal to another. [NIH]

Kinetics: The study of rate dynamics in chemical or physical systems. [NIH]

Leukopenia: A condition in which the number of leukocytes (white blood cells) in the blood is reduced. [NIH]

Lipid: Fat. [NIH]

Liver: A large, glandular organ located in the upper abdomen. The liver cleanses the blood and aids in digestion by secreting bile. [NIH]

Lumbar: Pertaining to the loins, the part of the back between the thorax and the pelvis. [EU]

MEDLINE: An online database of MEDLARS, the computerized bibliographic Medical Literature Analysis and Retrieval System of the National Library of Medicine. [NIH]

Membrane: A very thin layer of tissue that covers a surface. [NIH]

Memory: Complex mental function having four distinct phases: (1) memorizing or learning, (2) retention, (3) recall, and (4) recognition. Clinically, it is usually subdivided into immediate, recent, and remote memory. [NIH]

Meninges: The three membranes that cover and protect the brain and spinal cord. [NIH]

Mental: Pertaining to the mind; psychic. 2. (L. mentum chin) pertaining to the chin. [EU]

Mental Health: The state wherein the person is well adjusted. [NIH]

Mentors: Senior professionals who provide guidance, direction and support to those persons desirous of improvement in academic positions, administrative positions or other career development situations. [NIH]

Methotrexate: An antineoplastic antimetabolite with immunosuppressant properties. It is an inhibitor of dihydrofolate reductase and prevents the formation of tetrahydrofolate, necessary for synthesis of thymidylate, an essential component of DNA. [NIH]

MI: Myocardial infarction. Gross necrosis of the myocardium as a result of interruption of the blood supply to the area; it is almost always caused by atherosclerosis of the coronary arteries, upon which coronary thrombosis is usually superimposed. [NIH]

Mineralization: The action of mineralizing; the state of being mineralized. [EU]

Modification: A change in an organism, or in a process in an organism, that is acquired from its own activity or environment. [NIH]

Molecular: Of, pertaining to, or composed of molecules : a very small mass of matter. [EU]

Myocardium: The muscle tissue of the heart composed of striated, involuntary muscle known as cardiac muscle. [NIH]

Necrosis: A pathological process caused by the progressive degradative action of enzymes that is generally associated with severe cellular trauma. It is characterized by mitochondrial swelling, nuclear flocculation, uncontrolled cell lysis, and ultimately cell death. [NIH]

Nephropathy: Disease of the kidneys. [EU]

Nerve: A cordlike structure of nervous tissue that connects parts of the nervous system with other tissues of the body and conveys nervous impulses to, or away from, these tissues. [NIH]

Nervous System: The entire nerve apparatus composed of the brain, spinal cord, nerves and ganglia. [NIH]

Neurologic: Having to do with nerves or the nervous system. [NIH]

Neurotransmitter: Any of a group of substances that are released on excitation from the axon terminal of a presynaptic neuron of the central or peripheral nervous system and travel across the synaptic cleft to either excite or inhibit the target cell. Among the many substances that have the properties of a neurotransmitter are acetylcholine, norepinephrine, epinephrine, dopamine, glycine, y-aminobutyrate, glutamic acid, substance P, enkephalins, endorphins, and serotonin. [EU]

Neutrons: Electrically neutral elementary particles found in all atomic nuclei except light hydrogen; the mass is equal to that of the proton and electron combined and they are unstable when isolated from the nucleus, undergoing beta decay. Slow, thermal, epithermal, and fast neutrons refer to the energy levels with which the neutrons are ejected from heavier nuclei during their decay. [NIH]

On-line: A sexually-reproducing population derived from a common parentage. [NIH]

Orthopedics: A surgical specialty which utilizes medical, surgical, and physical methods to treat and correct deformities, diseases, and injuries to the skeletal system, its articulations, and associated structures. [NIH]

Osmosis: Tendency of fluids (e.g., water) to move from the less concentrated to the more concentrated side of a semipermeable membrane. [NIH]

Osteoblasts: Bone-forming cells which secrete an extracellular matrix. Hydroxyapatite crystals are then deposited into the matrix to form bone. [NIH]

Osteoclasts: A large multinuclear cell associated with the absorption and removal of bone. An odontoclast, also called cementoclast, is cytomorphologically the same as an osteoclast and is involved in cementum resorption. [NIH]

Osteodystrophy: Defective bone formation. [EU]

Osteogenic sarcoma: A malignant tumor of the bone. Also called osteosarcoma. [NIH]

Osteomalacia: A condition marked by softening of the bones (due to impaired mineralization, with excess accumulation of osteoid), with pain, tenderness, muscular weakness, anorexia, and loss of weight, resulting from deficiency of vitamin D and calcium. [EU]

Osteopathic Medicine: A system of therapy and medicine based on the theory that the normal body is a vital mechanical organism whose structural and functional states are of equal importance and is capable of making its own remedies against infections and toxic conditions when there are favorable environmental circumstances and adequate nutrition. [NIH]

Osteopetrosis: Excessive formation of dense trabecular bone leading to pathological fractures, osteitis, splenomegaly with infarct, anemia, and extramedullary hemopoiesis. [NIH]

Osteoporosis: Reduction of bone mass without alteration in the composition of bone, leading to fractures. Primary osteoporosis can be of two major types: postmenopausal osteoporosis and age-related (or senile) osteoporosis. [NIH]

Osteosarcoma: A cancer of the bone that affects primarily children and adolescents. Also called osteogenic sarcoma. [NIH]

Oxalate: A chemical that combines with calcium in urine to form the most common type of kidney stone (calcium oxalate stone). [NIH]

Pancreas: A mixed exocrine and endocrine gland situated transversely across the posterior abdominal wall in the epigastric and hypochondriac regions. The endocrine portion is comprised of the Islets of Langerhans, while the exocrine portion is a compound acinar gland that secretes digestive enzymes. [NIH]

Pancreas Transplant: A surgical procedure that involves replacing the pancreas of a person who has diabetes with a healthy pancreas that can make insulin. The healthy pancreas comes from a donor who has just died or from a living relative. A person can donate half a pancreas and still live normally. [NIH]

Pancreas Transplantation: The transference of a pancreas from one human or animal to another. [NIH]

Pathologic: 1. Indicative of or caused by a morbid condition. 2. Pertaining to pathology (= branch of medicine that treats the essential nature of the disease, especially the structural and functional changes in tissues and organs of the body caused by the disease). [EU]

Peptide: Any compound consisting of two or more amino acids, the building blocks of proteins. Peptides are combined to make proteins. [NIH]

Pericarditis: Inflammation of the pericardium. [EU]

Pharmacologic: Pertaining to pharmacology or to the properties and reactions of drugs. [EU]

Phosphorus: A non-metallic element that is found in the blood, muscles, nevers, bones, and teeth, and is a component of adenosine triphosphate (ATP; the primary energy source for the body's cells.) [NIH]

Plasma: The clear, yellowish, fluid part of the blood that carries the blood cells. The proteins that form blood clots are in plasma. [NIH]

Pneumonia: Inflammation of the lungs. [NIH]

Polypeptide: A peptide which on hydrolysis yields more than two amino acids; called tripeptides, tetrapeptides, etc. according to the number of amino acids contained. [EU]

Posterior: Situated in back of, or in the back part of, or affecting the back or dorsal surface of the body. In lower animals, it refers to the caudal end of the body. [EU]

Postmenopausal: Refers to the time after menopause. Menopause is the time in a woman's life when menstrual periods stop permanently; also called "change of life." [NIH]

Practice Guidelines: Directions or principles presenting current or future rules of policy for the health care practitioner to assist him in patient care decisions regarding diagnosis, therapy, or related clinical circumstances. The guidelines may be developed by government agencies at any level, institutions, professional societies, governing boards, or by the convening of expert panels. The guidelines form a basis for the evaluation of all aspects of health care and delivery. [NIH]

Progressive: Advancing; going forward; going from bad to worse; increasing in scope or severity. [EU]

Prophylaxis: An attempt to prevent disease. [NIH]

Protein C: A vitamin-K dependent zymogen present in the blood, which, upon activation by thrombin and thrombomodulin exerts anticoagulant properties by inactivating factors Va and VIIIa at the rate-limiting steps of thrombin formation. [NIH]

Protein Conformation: The characteristic 3-dimensional shape of a protein, including the secondary, supersecondary (motifs), tertiary (domains) and quaternary structure of the peptide chain. Quaternary protein structure describes the conformation assumed by multimeric proteins (aggregates of more than one polypeptide chain). [NIH]

Protein S: The vitamin K-dependent cofactor of activated protein C. Together with protein C, it inhibits the action of factors VIIIa and Va. A deficiency in protein S can lead to recurrent venous and arterial thrombosis. [NIH]

Proteins: Polymers of amino acids linked by peptide bonds. The specific sequence of amino acids determines the shape and function of the protein. [NIH]

Protons: Stable elementary particles having the smallest known positive charge, found in the nuclei of all elements. The proton mass is less than that of a neutron. A proton is the nucleus of the light hydrogen atom, i.e., the hydrogen ion. [NIH]

Psoriasis: A common genetically determined, chronic, inflammatory skin disease characterized by rounded erythematous, dry, scaling patches. The lesions have a predilection for nails, scalp, genitalia, extensor surfaces, and the lumbosacral region. Accelerated epidermopoiesis is considered to be the fundamental pathologic feature in psoriasis. [NIH]

Public Health: Branch of medicine concerned with the prevention and control of disease and disability, and the promotion of physical and mental health of the population on the international, national, state, or municipal level. [NIH]

Public Policy: A course or method of action selected, usually by a government, from among alternatives to guide and determine present and future decisions. [NIH]

Publishing: "The business or profession of the commercial production and issuance of literature" (Webster's 3d). It includes the publisher, publication processes, editing and editors. Production may be by conventional printing methods or by electronic publishing. [NIH]

Pulmonary: Relating to the lungs. [NIH]

Pulmonary Artery: The short wide vessel arising from the conus arteriosus of the right ventricle and conveying unaerated blood to the lungs. [NIH]

Radiation: Emission or propagation of electromagnetic energy (waves/rays), or the waves/rays themselves; a stream of electromagnetic particles (electrons, neutrons, protons, alpha particles) or a mixture of these. The most common source is the sun. [NIH]

Radiography: Examination of any part of the body for diagnostic purposes by means of roentgen rays, recording the image on a sensitized surface (such as photographic film). [NIH]

Randomized: Describes an experiment or clinical trial in which animal or human subjects are assigned by chance to separate groups that compare different treatments. [NIH]

Reaction Time: The time from the onset of a stimulus until the organism responds. [NIH]

Reductase: Enzyme converting testosterone to dihydrotestosterone. [NIH]

Refer: To send or direct for treatment, aid, information, de decision. [NIH]

Regimen: A treatment plan that specifies the dosage, the schedule, and the duration of treatment. [NIH]

Renal failure: Progressive renal insufficiency and uremia, due to irreversible and progressive renal glomerular tubular or interstitial disease. [NIH]

Rheumatism: A group of disorders marked by inflammation or pain in the connective tissue structures of the body. These structures include bone, cartilage, and fat. [NIH]

Rheumatoid: Resembling rheumatism. [EU]

Rheumatoid arthritis: A form of arthritis, the cause of which is unknown, although infection, hypersensitivity, hormone imbalance and psychologic stress have been suggested as possible causes. [NIH]

Ribosome: A granule of protein and RNA, synthesized in the nucleolus and found in the cytoplasm of cells. Ribosomes are the main sites of protein synthesis. Messenger RNA attaches to them and there receives molecules of transfer RNA bearing amino acids. [NIH]

Screening: Checking for disease when there are no symptoms. [NIH]

Senile: Relating or belonging to old age; characteristic of old age; resulting from infirmity of old age. [NIH]

Serum: The clear liquid part of the blood that remains after blood cells and clotting proteins have been removed. [NIH]

Skeletal: Having to do with the skeleton (boney part of the body). [NIH]

Skeleton: The framework that supports the soft tissues of vertebrate animals and protects many of their internal organs. The skeletons of vertebrates are made of bone and/or cartilage. [NIH]

Small intestine: The part of the digestive tract that is located between the stomach and the large intestine. [NIH]

Social Medicine: A branch of medicine concerned with the role of socio-environmental factors in the occurrence, prevention and treatment of disease. [NIH]

Social Support: Support systems that provide assistance and encouragement to individuals with physical or emotional disabilities in order that they may better cope. Informal social support is usually provided by friends, relatives, or peers, while formal assistance is provided by churches, groups, etc. [NIH]

Specialist: In medicine, one who concentrates on 1 special branch of medical science. [NIH]

Spinal cord: The main trunk or bundle of nerves running down the spine through holes in the spinal bone (the vertebrae) from the brain to the level of the lower back. [NIH]

Splenomegaly: Enlargement of the spleen. [NIH]

Stimulus: That which can elicit or evoke action (response) in a muscle, nerve, gland or other excitable issue, or cause an augmenting action upon any function or metabolic process. [NIH]

Stomach: An organ of digestion situated in the left upper quadrant of the abdomen between the termination of the esophagus and the beginning of the duodenum. [NIH]

Stress: Forcibly exerted influence; pressure. Any condition or situation that causes strain or tension. Stress may be either physical or psychologic, or both. [NIH]

Stress management: A set of techniques used to help an individual cope more effectively with difficult situations in order to feel better emotionally, improve behavioral skills, and often to enhance feelings of control. Stress management may include relaxation exercises, assertiveness training, cognitive restructuring, time management, and social support. It can be delivered either on a one-to-one basis or in a group format. [NIH]

Stroke: Sudden loss of function of part of the brain because of loss of blood flow. Stroke may be caused by a clot (thrombosis) or rupture (hemorrhage) of a blood vessel to the brain. [NIH]

Systemic: Affecting the entire body. [NIH]

Thigh: A leg; in anatomy, any elongated process or part of a structure more or less comparable to a leg. [NIH]

Thoracic: Having to do with the chest. [NIH]

Thyroid: A gland located near the windpipe (trachea) that produces thyroid hormone, which helps regulate growth and metabolism. [NIH]

Thyroid Gland: A highly vascular endocrine gland consisting of two lobes, one on either side of the trachea, joined by a narrow isthmus; it produces the thyroid hormones which are concerned in regulating the metabolic rate of the body. [NIH]

Tone: 1. The normal degree of vigour and tension; in muscle, the resistance to passive elongation or stretch; tonus. 2. A particular quality of sound or of voice. 3. To make permanent, or to change, the colour of silver stain by chemical treatment, usually with a heavy metal. [EU]

Toxic: Having to do with poison or something harmful to the body. Toxic substances usually cause unwanted side effects. [NIH]

Toxicology: The science concerned with the detection, chemical composition, and pharmacologic action of toxic substances or poisons and the treatment and prevention of toxic manifestations. [NIH]

Transfection: The uptake of naked or purified DNA into cells, usually eukaryotic. It is analogous to bacterial transformation. [NIH]

Translation: The process whereby the genetic information present in the linear sequence of ribonucleotides in mRNA is converted into a corresponding sequence of amino acids in a protein. It occurs on the ribosome and is unidirectional. [NIH]

Ultrafiltration: The separation of particles from a suspension by passage through a filter with very fine pores. In ultrafiltration the separation is accomplished by convective transport; in dialysis separation relies instead upon differential diffusion. Ultrafiltration occurs naturally and is a laboratory procedure. Artificial ultrafiltration of the blood is referred to as hemofiltration or hemodiafiltration (if combined with hemodialysis). [NIH]

Uremia: The illness associated with the buildup of urea in the blood because the kidneys are not working effectively. Symptoms include nausea, vomiting, loss of appetite, weakness, and mental confusion. [NIH]

Urine: Fluid containing water and waste products. Urine is made by the kidneys, stored in the bladder, and leaves the body through the urethra. [NIH]

Vaccines: Suspensions of killed or attenuated microorganisms (bacteria, viruses, fungi, protozoa, or rickettsiae), antigenic proteins derived from them, or synthetic constructs, administered for the prevention, amelioration, or treatment of infectious and other diseases. [NIH]

Veterinary Medicine: The medical science concerned with the prevention, diagnosis, and treatment of diseases in animals. [NIH]

Viral: Pertaining to, caused by, or of the nature of virus. [EU]

Virus: Submicroscopic organism that causes infectious disease. In cancer therapy, some viruses may be made into vaccines that help the body build an immune response to, and kill, tumor cells. [NIH]

Visceral: , from viscus a viscus) pertaining to a viscus. [EU]

Vitro: Descriptive of an event or enzyme reaction under experimental investigation occurring outside a living organism. Parts of an organism or microorganism are used together with artificial substrates and/or conditions. [NIH]

X-ray: High-energy radiation used in low doses to diagnose diseases and in high doses to treat cancer. [NIH]

INDEX

A

Abdominal, 61, 71
Algorithms, 61, 62
Alkaline, 7, 61, 62
Alpha Particles, 61, 72
Alternative medicine, 5, 27, 28, 61
Aluminum, 7, 8, 11, 61
Amino acid, 34, 35, 61, 67, 71, 72, 73, 74
Amino Acid Sequence, 34, 35, 61
Amyloid, 14, 61
Anaemia, 18, 61
Anemia, 61, 62, 70
Ankle, 9, 61
Anomalies, 61, 66
Anorexia, 61, 70
Anticonvulsant, 21, 62
Antimetabolite, 62, 69
Antineoplastic, 62, 69
Aorta, 62, 65
Arteries, 62, 64, 69
Arthropathy, 9, 19, 62
Articular, 34, 35, 62
Autopsy, 8, 62

B

Back Pain, 12, 14, 19, 62
Beta-pleated, 61, 62
Bewilderment, 62, 64
Bile, 62, 69
Biotechnology, 6, 45, 62
Blood Coagulation, 62, 63
Blood pressure, 62, 63, 68
Blood vessel, 62, 63, 73
Bone Resorption, 11, 62

C

Cadmium, 8, 11, 62
Cadmium Poisoning, 62
Calcitonin, 34, 62
Calcium, 8, 15, 21, 62, 63, 70, 71
Calcium Oxalate, 63, 71
Cardiac, 63, 67, 69
Cardiovascular, 4, 63
Cardiovascular disease, 4, 63
Cell, 4, 8, 62, 63, 64, 66, 69, 70
Cell Division, 63
Cell proliferation, 4, 63
Central Nervous System, 12, 63
Cerebrovascular, 63
Chiropractic, 3, 7, 16, 19, 28, 30, 63

Chronic, 11, 14, 19, 62, 63, 68, 72
Clinical trial, 4, 5, 45, 63, 72
Cloning, 62, 63
Cognitive restructuring, 63, 73
Collagen, 61, 63
Complement, 7, 63, 64
Complementary and alternative medicine, 27, 28, 31, 64
Complementary medicine, 7, 8, 28, 64
Computational Biology, 45, 64
Confusion, 17, 21, 64, 65, 74
Consciousness, 64, 65
Contraindications, ii, 64
Convulsions, 62, 64
Coronary, 63, 64, 69
Coronary heart disease, 63, 64
Coronary Thrombosis, 64, 69
Cortex, 64, 65
Cortical, 10, 65
Cranial, 9, 10, 11, 16, 28, 30, 65

D

Dehydration, 36, 65
Dementia, 4, 65
Dermis, 65, 66
Diabetes Mellitus, 8, 65, 67, 68
Diagnostic procedure, 33, 65
Dialyzer, 65, 67
Diffusion, 65, 67, 74
Digestion, 62, 65, 69, 73
Direct, iii, 65, 72
Disorientation, 64, 65
Distemper, 8, 65
Distemper Virus, Canine, 65
Dominance, 20, 65
Drive, ii, vi, 19, 23, 65
Ductus Arteriosus, 28, 65
Dyes, 61, 65

E

Efficacy, 28, 65
Electrolyte, 65, 67
Electrons, 66, 72
Endotoxins, 64, 66, 69
Environmental Health, 44, 46, 66
Enzymatic, 61, 63, 64, 66
Enzyme, 66, 68, 72, 74
Epigastric, 66, 71
Erythrocytes, 61, 66
Exocrine, 66, 71

Exostoses, 18, 66
Extensor, 66, 72
Extracellular, 61, 66, 70
Extracellular Matrix, 66, 70
F
Family Planning, 45, 66
Fat, 64, 66, 69, 72
Feline Panleukopenia, 65, 66
Femoral, 19, 66
Femur, 66
Fetal Blood, 65, 66
Focal Dermal Hypoplasia, 11, 66
G
Gastrectomy, 18, 66
Gastrin, 66, 67
Gastrointestinal, 62, 65, 67
Gene, 10, 62, 65, 67
Genetics, 65, 67
Geriatric, 4, 67
Gland, 67, 71, 73
Glomerular, 67, 72
Glucose, 65, 67, 68
Glucose Intolerance, 65, 67
Glycine, 61, 67, 70
Governing Board, 67, 71
H
Haemodialysis, 19, 67
Health Services, 10, 67
Heart attack, 63, 67
Hemodialysis, 11, 14, 15, 65, 67, 74
Hemofiltration, 8, 67, 74
Hepatic, 18, 67
Heredity, 67
Heterozygotes, 65, 67
Histology, 15, 67
Homozygotes, 65, 67
Hormone, 34, 62, 66, 67, 68, 72, 73
Hydroxyproline, 61, 63, 68
Hyperostosis, 10, 68
Hyperoxaluria, 18, 68
Hypersensitivity, 68, 72
Hypertension, 63, 68
Hyperthyroidism, 15, 68
Hypertrophy, 66, 68
Hypoplasia, 66, 68
I
Idiopathic, 12, 68
Idiosyncrasy, 11, 68
Immune response, 68, 74
Immunosuppressant, 68, 69
In vitro, 12, 68
In vivo, 68

Infarction, 64, 68, 69
Infection, 66, 68, 72
Inflammation, 65, 68, 71, 72
Ingestion, 62, 68
Insulin, 68, 71
Interstitial, 68, 72
Intestinal, 18, 21, 68
Intestines, 61, 67, 68
Intoxication, 11, 68
Isoenzyme, 7, 68
K
Kb, 44, 69
Keto, 18, 69
Kidney stone, 69, 71
Kidney Transplantation, 18, 69
Kinetics, 15, 34, 35, 69
L
Leukopenia, 65, 69
Lipid, 68, 69
Liver, 18, 61, 62, 67, 69
Lumbar, 62, 69
M
MEDLINE, 45, 69
Membrane, 64, 65, 66, 67, 69, 70
Memory, 61, 65, 69
Meninges, 63, 69
Mental, iv, 4, 44, 46, 64, 65, 69, 72, 74
Mental Health, iv, 4, 44, 46, 69, 72
Mentors, 4, 69
Methotrexate, 11, 12, 13, 15, 69
MI, 59, 69
Mineralization, 69, 70
Modification, 61, 69
Molecular, 45, 47, 62, 64, 69
Myocardium, 69
N
Necrosis, 68, 69
Nephropathy, 18, 70
Nerve, 63, 70, 73
Nervous System, 63, 70
Neurologic, 65, 70
Neurotransmitter, 61, 67, 70
Neutrons, 61, 70, 72
O
On-line, 27, 59, 70
Orthopedics, 9, 10, 40, 70
Osmosis, 36, 70
Osteoblasts, 34, 35, 70
Osteoclasts, 62, 70
Osteodystrophy, 18, 70
Osteogenic sarcoma, 70
Osteomalacia, 18, 70

Osteopathic Medicine, 3, 70
Osteopetrosis, 8, 70
Osteoporosis, 34, 50, 70
Osteosarcoma, 13, 70
Oxalate, 18, 68, 71
P
Pancreas, 19, 61, 68, 71
Pancreas Transplant, 19, 71
Pancreas Transplantation, 19, 71
Pathologic, 10, 64, 68, 71, 72
Peptide, 34, 35, 61, 62, 71, 72
Pericarditis, 19, 71
Pharmacologic, 28, 71, 74
Phosphorus, 63, 71
Plasma, 62, 67, 71
Pneumonia, 24, 64, 71
Polypeptide, 61, 63, 71, 72
Posterior, 62, 71
Postmenopausal, 70, 71
Practice Guidelines, 46, 71
Progressive, 10, 65, 69, 71, 72
Prophylaxis, 18, 71
Protein C, 61, 71
Protein Conformation, 61, 71
Protein S, 62, 71, 72, 73
Proteins, 61, 63, 71, 72, 73, 74
Protons, 61, 72
Psoriasis, 13, 72
Public Health, 4, 5, 46, 72
Public Policy, 45, 72
Publishing, 6, 72
Pulmonary, 62, 65, 67, 72
Pulmonary Artery, 62, 65, 72
R
Radiation, 17, 72, 74
Radiography, 7, 72
Randomized, 65, 72
Reaction Time, 36, 72
Reductase, 69, 72
Refer, 1, 63, 70, 72
Regimen, 65, 72
Renal failure, 20, 72
Rheumatism, 8, 72
Rheumatoid, 13, 72

Rheumatoid arthritis, 13, 72
Ribosome, 73, 74
S
Screening, 63, 73
Senile, 70, 73
Serum, 7, 63, 73
Skeletal, 13, 18, 20, 70, 73
Skeleton, 66, 73
Small intestine, 67, 68, 73
Social Medicine, 4, 73
Social Support, 73
Specialist, 51, 73
Spinal cord, 63, 69, 70, 73
Splenomegaly, 70, 73
Stimulus, 65, 72, 73
Stomach, 61, 66, 67, 68, 73
Stress, 19, 39, 72, 73
Stress management, 39, 73
Stroke, 44, 63, 73
Systemic, 8, 62, 68, 73
T
Thigh, 66, 73
Thoracic, 62, 73
Thyroid, 62, 68, 73
Thyroid Gland, 68, 73
Tone, 74
Toxic, iv, 70, 74
Toxicology, 46, 74
Transfection, 62, 74
Translation, 5, 61, 74
U
Ultrafiltration, 67, 74
Uremia, 72, 74
Urine, 63, 68, 69, 71, 74
V
Vaccines, 74
Veterinary Medicine, 45, 74
Viral, 65, 74
Virus, 8, 65, 66, 74
Visceral, 34, 35, 74
Vitro, 74
X
X-ray, 9, 21, 74

Printed in the United Kingdom
by Lightning Source UK Ltd.
118842UK00001B/76